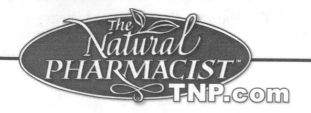

Inside—Find the Answers to These Questions and More

☑ What is policosanol, and how does it compare to statin drugs? (See page 74.)

☑ What are stanols, and how can they lower cholesterol levels? (See page 67.)

☑ Does soy interact with any medications? (See page 73.)

☑ How effective is red yeast rice for lowering my cholesterol? (See page 77.)

☑ Is garlic effective for high cholesterol? (See page 18.)

☑ Will garlic reduce my high blood pressure? (See page 27.)

☑ What medications should I not combine with garlic? (See page 46.)

☑ What are the benefits and risks of niacin? (See page 53.)

☑ Can pantethine lower my triglyceride levels? (See page 86.)

☑ What dietary changes might be helpful to improve my cholesterol levels? (See page 100.)

P9-CQH-797

The Natural Pharmacist™ Library

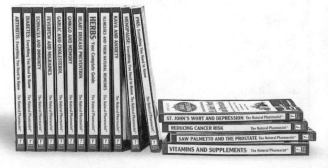

Visit us online at www.TNP.com

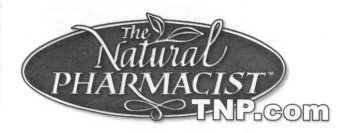

Lowering
Cholesterol

Darin Ingels, N.D.

Series Editors
Steven Bratman, M.D.
David Kroll, Ph.D.

A DIVISION OF PRIMA PUBLISHING

Visit us online at www.TNP.com

Special thanks to Drs. Brammer, Dipasquale,
Lamden and Donovan, Jon Goodman, Melissa Macfarlane,
Susie Wickstead, my families, and especially my wife,
Michelle, for her love and support.

Warning—Disclaimer

This book is not intended to provide medical advice and is sold with the understanding that the publisher and the author are not liable for the misconception or misuse of information provided. The author and Prima Publishing shall have neither liability nor responsibility to any person or entity with respect to any loss, damage, or injury caused or alleged to be caused directly or indirectly by the information contained in this book or the use of any products mentioned. Readers should not use any of the products discussed in this book without the advice of a medical professional.

The Food and Drug Administration has not approved the use of any of the natural treatments discussed in this book. This book and the information contained herein, has not been approved by the Food and Drug Administration.

Pseudonyms are used throughout to protect the privacy of individuals involved.

PRIMA HEALTH and colophon are trademarks of Prima Communications, Inc. THE NATURAL PHARMACIST™ is a trademark of Prima Communications, Inc.

Illustrations by Helene D. Stevens and Gale Mueller.
Illustrations © 1999 Prima Publishing. All rights reserved.

All products mentioned in this book are trademarks of their respective companies.

Library of Congress Cataloging-in-Publication Data on file
ISBN 0-7615-1555-0

01 02 03 04 HH 10 9 8 7
Printed in the United States of America

Visit us online at www.TNP.com

Contents

Contents

What Makes This Book Different?

The interest in natural medicine has never been greater. According to the National Association of Chain Drug Stores, 65 million Americans are using natural supplements, and the number is growing! Yet it is hard for the consumer to find trustworthy sources for balanced information about this emerging field. Why? Frankly, natural medicine has had a checkered history. From snake oil potions sold at the turn of the century to those books, magazines, and product catalogs that hype miracle cures today, this is a field where exaggerated claims have been the norm. Proponents of natural medicine have tended to abuse science, treating it more as a marketing tool than a means of discovering the truth.

But there is truth to be found. Studies of vitamins, minerals, and other food supplements have been with us since these nutritional substances were first discovered, and the level and quality of this science has grown dramatically in the last 20 years. Herbal medicine has been neglected in the United States, but in Europe, this, the oldest of all healing arts, has been the subject of tremendous and ongoing scientific interest.

At present, for a number of herbs and supplements, it is possible to give reasonably scientific answers to the following questions: How well does this work? How safe is it? What types of conditions is it best used for?

THE NATURAL PHARMACIST series is designed to cut through the hype and tell you what we know and what remains to be researched regarding popular natural treatments. These books are more conservative than any others available, more honest about the weaknesses of natural approaches, more fair in their comparisons of natural and conventional treatments. You won't find any miracle cures here, but you will discover useful options that can help you become healthier.

Why Choose Natural Treatments?

Although the science behind natural medicine continues to grow, this is still a much less scientifically validated field than conventional medicine. You might ask, "Why should I resort to an herb that is only partly proven, when I could take a drug with solid science behind it?" There are at least three good reasons to consider natural alternatives.

First, some herbs and supplements offer benefits that are not matched by any conventional drug. Echinacea is a good example. If you have a cold and take echinacea, you'll recover faster. No standard medication can do the same.

Another example is glucosamine sulfate for arthritis. Glucosamine seems to slow the progression of arthritis, meaning that it protects your joints from getting worse over time. There is no pill or tablet your doctor can prescribe that offers the same benefit.

In many cases, the science behind natural treatments is very strong. For example, there is more evidence for the herb St. John's wort than there was for Prozac when it was first approved as a drug. The science behind other natural treatments is less than perfect, but when the risks are low and the possible benefit high, a natural treatment may be worth trying. It is a little-known fact that for many conventional treatments the science is less than perfect as well, and physicians must balance uncertain benefits against incompletely understood risks.

A second reason to consider natural therapies is that some may offer benefits comparable to those of drugs with fewer side effects. Again, the herb St. John's wort is a good example. Scientific evidence suggests that this herb is just as effective for mild to moderate depression as standard drugs, while producing fewer side effects. Saw palmetto for benign enlargement of the prostate, ginkgo for relieving symptoms and perhaps slowing the progression of Alzheimer's disease, and chondroitin for osteoarthritis are other examples. This is not to say that herbs and supplements are completely harmless—they're not—but for most the level of risk is quite low. The biggest potential problems are interactions between drugs and herbs, and we cover these thoroughly in our books.

Finally, there is a philosophical point to consider. For many people, it "feels" better to use a treatment that comes from nature instead of from a laboratory. Just as you might rather wear all-cotton clothing than polyester or look at a mountain landscape rather than the skyscrapers of a downtown city, natural treatments may simply feel more compatible with your view of life. We can quibble endlessly about just what "natural" means and whether a certain treatment is "actually" natural or not, but such arguments are beside the point. The difference is in the feeling, and feelings matter. In fact, having a good feeling about taking an herb may lead you to use it more consistently than you would a prescription drug.

Of course, at times synthetic drugs may be necessary and even lifesaving. But on many other occasions it may be quite reasonable to turn to an herb or supplement instead of a drug.

To make good decisions you need good information. Unfortunately, while hundreds of books on alternative medicine are published every year, many are highly misleading. The phrase "studies prove" is often used when the studies in question are so small or so badly conducted that they prove nothing at all. You may even find that the "data" from other books comes from studies with petri dishes and not real people!

You can't even assume that books written by well-known authors are scientifically sound. Many of these authors rely on secondary writers, leading to a game of "telephone," where misconceptions are passed around from book to book. And there's a strong tendency to exaggerate the power of natural remedies, whitewashing them with selective reporting.

THE NATURAL PHARMACIST series gives you the balanced information you need to make informed decisions about your health needs. Setting a new, high standard of accuracy and objectivity, these books take a realistic look at the herbs and supplements you read about in the news. You will encounter both favorable and unfavorable studies in these pages and will learn about both the benefits and the risks of natural treatments.

THE NATURAL PHARMACIST series is the source you can trust.

Steven Bratman, M.D.
David Kroll, Ph.D.

Introduction

If you asked most people on the street what the greatest health concern facing America is right now, you might get answers such as "cancer" or "AIDS." What many don't realize is cardiovascular disease is the number one killer in the developed world. In America alone, over 58 million people suffer from such problems as angina, heart attacks, strokes, and aortic aneurysm, and almost 1 million die each year as a consequence.

While there are many causes of cardiovascular disease, high cholesterol is undoubtedly one of the most important. Unfortunately, high cholesterol by itself does not usually cause symptoms. In fact, the symptoms may not become apparent until the onset of crushing chest pain, and the arrival of an ambulance to take you to intensive care. This is one disease that you must identify early, to spare yourself avoidable risk and suffering.

Interestingly, physicians did not at first realize that high cholesterol levels were cause for concern. Actually, for a while, they thought low cholesterol was the cause of heart attacks. This misconception came about because right after a heart attack, the measured cholesterol level is unusually low. The breakthrough came after the residents of Framingham, Massachusetts, agreed to participate in an enormous long-term study that continues to the present day. It was this Framingham study that woke up the medical world to the risks presented by high cholesterol levels in the blood. Because of Framingham, by the late 1950s, we could no longer eat a breakfast consisting of sausage, bacon, eggs fried in lard, and white toast liberally smeared with butter without imagining clumps of fat sticking to our arteries. The lowfat movement had begun.

Besides dietary changes, medical researchers began to search for treatments that could reduce cholesterol levels. The vitamin niacin was one of the earliest successful treatments, followed by several different classes of medications. In the 1980s, an advanced type of drug called HMG-CoA reductase inhibitors, or statin drugs, became available. These drugs are capable of specifically reducing cholesterol production with few side effects. Both niacin and statin drugs have been shown to save lives.

Besides niacin, there are numerous natural options for lowering cholesterol as well.

Garlic is one of the most famous natural treatments for high cholesterol, and in this book we cover it more extensively than any other herb or supplement. It does appear to be effective, but only modestly. Garlic won't lower your cholesterol very much. However, it has many positive effects, and, when these are combined, the overall heart-health benefit appears to be significant.

Stanol esters are a new and highly effective treatment for high cholesterol. These are added to certain margarines and other foods found in the grocery store. Stanols can significantly lower cholesterol by themselves; in addition, if you are taking statin drugs and still need to lower your cholesterol further, stanol-supplemented foods can help.

Soy products have also been found to reduce cholesterol. The evidence is so strong that the FDA has allowed manufacturers of soy products to write "heart healthy" on the label.

Although less well known than some of these other natural treatments, the supplement policosanol also appears to be quite effective for improving cholesterol levels. The Chinese food red yeast rice contains naturally occurring substances in the statin drug family, and for this reason it appears to lower cholesterol significantly.

Other natural treatments that might also help include guggul, chitosan, artichoke leaf, pantethine, and fish oil. High-fiber foods, certain oils, and nuts also appear to reduce cholesterol levels.

This book will fairly examine all the options (including conventional treatment), helping you to decide what approach is best for you.

Atherosclerosis and High Cholesterol

There is only one reason for you to lower your cholesterol: high cholesterol levels cause atherosclerosis. In this chapter, we'll present background information on atherosclerosis and its relationship to cholesterol, which you might find helpful when reading the later chapters. If you wish to start right in with natural treatments for high cholesterol, please just take a glance at the sidebar, Types of Cholesterol, and skip ahead to the next chapter.

Atherosclerosis is a disorder of the larger arteries in the body that leads to thickening and hardening of the arterial wall, and deposits of a fatty substance known as *plaque*. It is the leading cause of death in men over the age of 35 and of all people over the age of 45. Atherosclerosis and its related diseases cause approximately 50% of all deaths in the United States.[1]

Atherosclerosis in the arteries that feed the heart (the coronary arteries) diminishes the flow of blood to the heart muscle (see figure 1), causing a type of pain known

Types of Cholesterol

LDL:	low-density lipoprotein; the unhealthy kind of cholesterol
Lipoprotein(a):	possibly the worst kind of LDL cholesterol
HDL:	high-density lipoprotein; the healthy form of cholesterol
Triglycerides:	fatty substances that may also be harmful

as *angina*. Blood clots also tend to form along the walls of the arteries in the heart. The clots may break free and lodge themselves across the width of the vessel, completely blocking the flow of blood. The part of the heart muscle that is fed by that artery then dies from lack of oxygen. Such blockage of the artery is commonly called a heart attack. (A similar process can occur in the blood vessels that feed the brain, leading to a stroke.)

Atherosclerosis can also weaken the wall of a major artery, causing it to enlarge (becoming an aneurysm), leak blood, and eventually rupture. Atherosclerosis in the arteries of the legs causes pain with mild exercise, a condition known as *intermittent claudication*. Other consequences of atherosclerosis include kidney disease and impotence.

Obviously, atherosclerosis is a disease that requires serious medical attention; left untreated, its consequences are serious. The good news is that atherosclerosis can be prevented and—even better—there is reasonably good evidence that it can even be *reversed* by eliminating the factors that cause it.

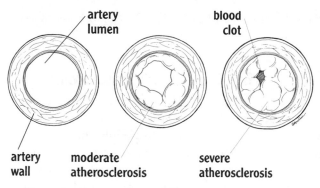

Figure 1. *Cross-section of three coronary arteries*

Risk Factors for Atherosclerosis

In 1948, a historic medical research project began. Known as the Framingham Heart Study, it aimed to follow the lives of 5,209 people living in Framingham, Massachusetts, for 30 years. The results have led to major changes in the lifestyles of many Americans, and indeed people all over the world. The Framingham study forever changed our view of food, turning the once-innocent pleasure of a breakfast of bacon and eggs, coffee with cream, and thickly buttered toast into a dangerous luxury.

The Framingham researchers found four major risk factors for atherosclerosis: high cholesterol in the blood, cigarette smoking, high blood pressure, and diabetes. Other probable risk factors include a sedentary lifestyle, a diet high in animal fats, being male, a family history of early heart disease, and high blood levels of homocysteine. (Homocysteine is a chemical in the blood that might accelerate atherosclerosis.)

This book will primarily address the first of these risk factors—high levels of cholesterol and related fatty substances in the blood. For more detailed information about the other risk factors, see THE NATURAL PHARMACIST book on heart disease prevention.

What Causes Atherosclerosis?

Despite decades of intensive study, we still do not fully understand the causes of atherosclerosis, although we do know a great deal. Contrary to popular belief, cholesterol doesn't simply accumulate in arteries the way grease builds up in pipes. Rather, the process involves progressive damage to the lining of arteries, in which cholesterol plays only a contributing role.

Although symptoms don't appear until adulthood, atherosclerosis comes on slowly, beginning early in childhood

The good news is that atherosclerosis can be prevented and there is reasonably good evidence that it can even be reversed by eliminating the factors that cause it.

and only gradually progressing to full-scale disease. Several studies have shown that signs of atherosclerosis can be found in children as young as 1 year old and that by age 10 almost all children have fatty streaks in their blood vessels.[2,3]

Fatty streaks are flat, yellow spots in the artery wall, which can grow up to 1 centimeter or longer. Because they are flat, fatty streaks don't obstruct the blood vessel or disrupt blood flow. However, over time they can gradually develop into full-scale atherosclerosis. The leading theory regarding how this occurs is the "response to injury" hypothesis. According to this theory, atherosclerosis is first triggered by an injury to the inner lining of the arterial wall (the *endothelium*). What can cause such an injury? The endothelium can be injured by direct physical strain, such as high blood pressure. Also, irritating substances circulating in the blood can cause damage. Some of the suspected irritants in the blood include low-density lipoprotein molecules (also called LDL or "bad" cholesterol), homocysteine, glucose, and free radicals. (We will discuss LDL cholesterol in greater depth later in this chapter.) Atherosclerosis tends to develop especially quickly at forks in the blood vessels, probably because the current of blood strikes those areas with particular force.

Once the endothelium has been damaged, a type of white blood cell adheres to the site of injury, then works its way deeper into the arterial wall. There, it is trans-formed into a scavenger cell called a *macrophage.* Macro-phages collect molecules of cholesterol and other fatty substances until they are so fat-filled they look like micro-scopic fatty snowballs. At the same time, platelets (cells that normally circulate in the bloodstream waiting to re-pair leaks in blood vessels) begin to stick to the damaged artery wall and form a plug. When they do this, they also release several chemicals that cause muscle cells to mi-grate to the area. These muscle cells then reproduce, yielding fibrous substances and thickening the fatty streak.

Over time, more white blood cells arrive, and a growing collection of dead cells, fat, calcium, and fibrous tissue makes the artery wall swell. Eventually, the swelling reaches a size where it is called a *fibrous plaque.* Individual fibrous plaques subsequently connect to form what is called *complicated plaque.* Complicated plaque continues to grow in both size and thickness until the *lumen* (open space) of the artery becomes partially or completely blocked, or until the artery wall becomes so weak that it ruptures. Pieces of plaque can also break free from the vessel wall, creating small bleeding spots. The body responds by forming a blood clot to stop the bleeding. Clots may also form simply

When plaque restricts the flow of blood, symptoms such as angina, intermittent claudication, and temporary strokes (called TIAs) can result.

because the plaque's surface is ragged. Such *thrombi,* as the clots are called, can become integrated into the plaque or, even worse, break off and completely obstruct the artery somewhere downstream. Broken off bits of plaque can also do this.

When plaque narrows the open space in the blood vessel and restricts the flow of blood, symptoms such as angina, intermittent claudication, and temporary strokes called *transient ischemic attacks* (TIAs) can result. However, outright blockage of the blood vessel by a blood clot or a piece of plaque can lead to full-blown strokes and heart attacks.

The Link Between High Cholesterol and Atherosclerosis

Although, as we've just seen, cholesterol doesn't clog arteries directly, there is absolutely no doubt that high cholesterol is a major cause of atherosclerosis. In the Framingham and other large studies, elevated levels of blood cholesterol have been associated with as much as a 300% increase in the rate of death due to heart attacks. The higher the blood cholesterol levels, the greater the heart attack rate. Furthermore, in animal studies where high levels of cholesterol were induced, atherosclerosis has been found to develop at a greatly increased rate.

According to the American Heart Association, as many as 97 million Americans have elevated blood cholesterol levels, with almost 38 million adults exceeding levels defined as "high risk." Clearly, controlling your cholesterol level is one of the most important health-affirming steps you can take.

What Is Cholesterol?

Cholesterol is a kind of *lipid,* or fat, in the body. Although cholesterol plays a role in atherosclerosis, it is also an essential substance in the body. The body uses it to make bile, which we use to digest fats, as well as to produce vitamin D and hormones such as estrogen, progesterone, and testosterone.

The body directly manufactures about two-thirds of its total cholesterol. The other third comes into the body through food, primarily from animal products such as meat, milk, and eggs. Most cells in the body can make cholesterol, but more than 90% is created in the liver and the walls of the intestine.

Lipoproteins: "Good" Cholesterol Versus "Bad" Cholesterol

As a fat, cholesterol isn't water soluble, so it doesn't dissolve in the blood. To allow it to move around the body, a special carrier molecule known as a *lipoprotein* attaches to it. Lipoproteins have the capacity to help fats dissolve in water. They shuttle cholesterol and triglycerides between the different tissues of the body. (Triglycerides are discussed in more detail later in this section.) There are several different types of lipoprotein/cholesterol packages, and each has its own effect on the body. The major types are called low-density lipoprotein (LDL), high-density lipoprotein (HDL), and very low-density lipoprotein (VLDL). LDL appears to be the most harmful type and, therefore, is often referred to as "bad" cholesterol. Studies show that higher LDL levels are directly associated with accelerated atherosclerosis. Conversely, HDL is regarded as the "good" cholesterol, because higher levels of it are associated with a lower incidence of atherosclerosis. HDL's job appears to be carrying cholesterol from the tissues back to the liver for redistribution or elimination.

According to the American Heart Association, as many as 97 million Americans have elevated blood cholesterol levels, with almost 38 million adults exceeding levels defined as "high risk."

A special form of LDL called lipoprotein(a) may be even more harmful than regular LDL.[4,5] High levels of lipoprotein(a) have been associated with a tenfold increase in the risk for heart disease, regardless of total cholesterol and LDL levels. Lipoprotein(a) contains an additional protein that increases its ability to stick to the artery wall, apparently increasing its capacity to cause damage.

If HDL (high-density lipoprotein) is "good" cholesterol and LDL (low-density lipoprotein) is "bad" cholesterol, one would think that VLDL (very low-density lipoprotein) is "very bad" cholesterol. However, this isn't the case. Here's why: Instead of cholesterol, VLDL primarily contains other fatty substances called *triglycerides*. Triglycerides are not as harmful as cholesterol, although they too may accelerate atherosclerosis.

How Do I Know If I Have High Cholesterol?

Your doctor can determine your total blood cholesterol, HDL, and triglyceride levels with a blood test called a *lipid profile.* A mathematical calculation can then determine your LDL level as well. (VLDL levels are not usually reported, because total blood triglyceride levels are more relevant.) Because a fatty or high-cholesterol meal can temporarily raise your cholesterol level, you need to get your blood drawn for a lipid profile in the morning before you've eaten.

The United States' National Cholesterol Education Program currently recommends a goal of total cholesterol below 200 mg/dL (milligrams per deciliter). Total cholesterol levels between 200 and 240 mg/dL are considered to be borderline high; levels above 240 mg/dL are considered high risk. These levels are important not only as indicators of risk of heart disease, but also as a guideline to help you and your doctor choose among available therapies. Optimally, LDL ("bad" cholesterol) levels should be below 130 mg/dL, and HDL ("good" cholesterol) levels should be greater than 30 mg/dL. Triglyceride levels should be less than 250 mg/dL, and lipoprotein(a) levels should ideally fall below 20 mg/dL.

Another useful piece of information for determining your risk is the ratio between your total cholesterol level and HDL level, as well as the ratio between your HDL and LDL levels. These ratios are often called *cardiac risk factors* because they too relate to your risk of heart disease. The total cholesterol-to-HDL ratio should be no greater than 4.5:1, and the LDL-to-HDL ratio should not exceed 2.5:1. Higher ratios indicate a moderate to high risk, with the risk increasing as the ratio increases.

These values and ratios are tools that you and your doctor can use to assess your risk for atherosclerosis and cardiovascular disease. Studies have shown that for every 1% drop in total cholesterol there is a 2% decrease in the risk of having a heart attack. The risk for heart attack drops even more—by as much as 4%—when HDL levels increase by 1%.

Dave's Story

Dave was a 26-year-old man who came to the clinic at his wife's insistence. When asked why she wanted him to come in so badly, he said she was concerned about his weight. Although he didn't look obese, Dave was about 25 pounds overweight for his height.

During the course of the interview with his doctor, Dave revealed that his father had died of a heart attack at a young age and that his grandfather had also died young as a result of a stroke. Dave worked long hours as a computer analyst, so he only had the chance to eat one meal a day (which was always fast food), and he rarely exercised.

Dave had not been examined or given a blood test for many years. His doctor pointed out that he had many risk factors for heart disease: sedentary lifestyle, high-fat diet, and family history. To see if he had other risk factors, the doctor checked Dave's blood pressure and evaluated his cholesterol levels.

Dave's blood pressure turned out to be okay. However, his total cholesterol was 256 mg/dL (too high), his LDL cholesterol was 151 mg/dL (also too high), and his HDL was 25

How Do I Know If I Have Atherosclerosis?

A major problem in diagnosing atherosclerosis is that there are usually no symptoms until it is fairly advanced. In the arteries of the heart, blockage can reach up to 90% before you begin to feel chest pain. Sometimes with a

mg/dL (too low). These readings got Dave's attention. His doctor reassured him that he was probably not in any immediate danger, because he was still young, and that he had plenty of time to lower his cholesterol and make lifestyle changes before any complications arose.

They worked out a plan whereby Dave could gradually improve his diet and increase his level of exercise. The doctor had done some research on stanol esters, and he suggested that Dave could use a stanol-enriched margarine spread twice a day.

After 3 months, Dave returned for a reevaluation. He had dropped almost 15 pounds, and he said that he felt great. His total cholesterol had fallen to 206 mg/dL, his LDL cholesterol had dropped to 122 mg/dL, and his HDL cholesterol had risen to 35 mg/dL. It was a dramatic improvement.

Which helped most, the lifestyle changes or the stanols? It's hard to say. But in chapter 4, we present the evidence that shows us that stanols can have a positive impact on lipid levels.

stethoscope, it is possible to hear a sound made by blood passing through a narrowed artery. This sound, technically called a *bruit* (pronounced BREW-ee), is usually medium-pitched, with a blowing quality to it. A physician can also feel for a vibration called a *thrill*. However, you really want to catch atherosclerosis before it reaches this point. If your doctor suspects you have a significant amount of atherosclerosis, there are several technologically advanced tools that can reveal how much blockage has occurred. Diagnostic imaging such as Doppler studies (similar to the Doppler radar used for weather forecasting), catheterization, x ray, and CT scans may be used, depending on which particular arteries are affected and the type of information your doctor wants. Obviously, the best plan is to assess your risk factors for atherosclerosis and to get examined now rather than waiting until the condition has set in. Subsequent chapters will explain how you can do this.

A major problem in diagnosing atherosclerosis is that there are usually no symptoms until it is fairly advanced.

QUICK
REVIEW

- Atherosclerosis is a leading cause of death in the United States, resulting in strokes, heart attacks, and many other complications.
- Atherosclerosis causes damage to the arteries of the body and leads to decreased blood flow as well as a greater likelihood that blood clots or other obstructions will completely cut off the flow within a blood vessel.

- Although we don't know for certain what causes atherosclerosis, cholesterol plays a key role by damaging the artery wall.

- The two most important types of cholesterol are LDL (low-density lipoprotein, also known as "bad" cholesterol) and HDL (high-density lipoprotein, also called "good" cholesterol).

- In order to prevent atherosclerosis, it is important to have a regular lipid profile performed. This is a blood test that determines your total blood cholesterol level and your levels of HDL, LDL, and triglycerides.

CHAPTER
T W O

Garlic and High Cholesterol

T he herb garlic *(Allium sativum)* is one of the most famous natural treatments for reducing cholesterol. While other natural or synthetic treatments for high cholesterol are more powerful, garlic seems to offer a range of heart-healthy benefits that work together.

Garlic is a familiar sight at the grocery store, where you can find not only garlic powder, garlic salt, pickled and minced garlic, but whole fresh garlic in the produce section (see figure 2). This popular herb has been used as both a food and medicine by cultures worldwide for more than 5,000 years. Today, more than 2 million *tons* of garlic are grown each year!

Garlic gets much of its strong odor from sulfur. The herb contains a considerable amount of sulfur, in the form of several different chemical compounds. Garlic's major sulfur-containing ingredient, *alliin,* is relatively odorless. However, crushing or cutting garlic brings an enzyme called *allinase* into contact with alliin, producing a powerfully aromatic substance called *allicin.*

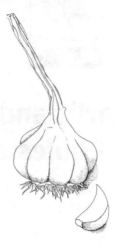

Figure 2. *Garlic*

You can see (or rather, *smell*) this chemical reaction at work with this simple experiment: Carefully peel a clove of fresh garlic, without scraping or cutting into the clove. Sniff the clove. Then smash it with the flat part of a knife and sniff again. The powerful odor released after the clove has been smashed lets you know that alliin and allinase have combined to produce allicin.

In addition to giving garlic most of its strong odor, allicin can blister the skin and kill bacteria, viruses, and fungi. Presumably, the garlic plant uses allicin and other sulfur compounds to protect itself from harmful microbes and insects. Allicin also appears to be at least partly responsible for garlic's anticholesterol effects. In addition, allicin quickly breaks down into other chemical compounds that may also contribute to garlic's medicinal properties.

Many researchers, in fact, believe that allicin is garlic's primary active ingredient. This is because laboratory research has found that allicin chemically inhibits enzymes responsible for making cholesterol. Furthermore, some garlic products that do not contain alliin have not proven effective in clinical studies. Other experts, however, disagree with the belief that allicin is the primary active ingredient.

Garlic also contains many chemical compounds that do not include sulfur. These compounds include several B vitamins, minerals, flavonoids, various amino acids, proteins, lipids, steroids, and 12 trace elements. These compounds contribute to the growth and life of the garlic plant, but we don't know whether they play a role in lowering cholesterol.

> **Garlic has been used as both a food and medicine by cultures worldwide for more than 5,000 years.**

The Possible Health Benefits of Garlic

Germany's Commission E is an official government agency that performs a job similar to that of the U.S. Food and Drug Administration (FDA), only it's specifically focused on herbs. In 1988 the commission authorized the use of garlic preparations "as an adjunct to dietary measures in patients with elevated blood lipids and for the prevention of age-related vascular changes." Stated simply, garlic is used to lower cholesterol and prevent hardening of the arteries.

Garlic appears to have a beneficial effect on several risk factors for atherosclerosis. It may reduce high blood pressure, "thin" the blood, and fight free radicals. These effects combined appear to lead to overall benefits against atherosclerosis.

Garlic and Cholesterol: The Scientific Evidence

One of the best and certainly the largest study on the effectiveness of garlic for high cholesterol was conducted in Germany and results were published in 1990.[1] Called the Mader study after its principal researcher, its results strongly suggest that regular use of garlic can lower cholesterol levels by an average of 12%. Although not perfect, the study was well designed, properly reported, and definitely worth taking seriously.

The Mader study was a double-blind placebo-controlled trial. This is the best and most reliable form of research. A treatment cannot really be considered proven effective unless it has been examined in properly designed and sufficiently large studies of this type.

The Mader study results strongly suggest that regular use of garlic can lower cholesterol levels by an average of 12%.

In a double-blind placebo-controlled trial, one group of participants receives the "real thing"—the active substance being tested. The other participants receive a placebo designed to appear, as much as possible, like the real thing. Neither group knows whether it's getting the real treatment or placebo (they are "blind"). Furthermore, the researchers administering placebo and real treatment are also kept in the dark about which group is receiving which treatment (making it a "double-blind" experiment). This last part is important, because it prevents the researchers from unintentionally tipping off the study participants or unconsciously biasing their evaluation of the results.

The purpose of this kind of study is to eliminate the power of suggestion. It is true, although hard to believe, that *placebo* (fake) treatments can produce dramatic and long-lasting results in a majority of the people who are given them. If the people in the real treatment group fare significantly better, it is a strong indication that the treatment really works.

The Mader Study

The Mader study enrolled 261 individuals selected from 30 different medical offices. Participants were randomly divided into two groups. One of the groups was given placebo. The other received four 200-mg garlic tablets each day. The garlic used in this study was a powder form standardized to contain 1.3% alliin. At the beginning of the study, participants had total cholesterol levels that averaged about 265 mg/dL, significantly higher than what is considered healthy. Cholesterol levels were measured every month for 4 months.

The results as they developed over this time period were impressive. In the group that received garlic, there was a steady decline in total cholesterol with each blood sample, but there was little change in the placebo group. At the end of 4 months, cholesterol levels in the garlic group had fallen from an average of about 265 mg/dL to 235 mg/dL, a 12% improvement. By comparison, there was only a 3% improvement in the placebo group. Triglyceride levels also fell significantly—by 17% in the treated group, as compared to only 2% in the placebo group. (See figure 3.)

Whenever you see good results in a study like this, you have to ask one question: Were the results statistically significant? That is, do they really mean anything, or could they have happened by chance? If you flip a coin 20 times and it comes up heads 14 times, you can't really conclude

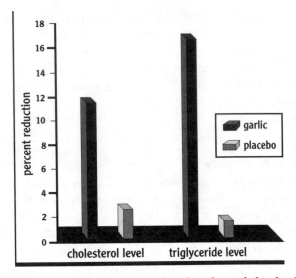

Figure 3. *Reduction in cholesterol and triglyceride levels after 4 months in a double-blind study* (Mader, 1990)

from this that the coin is biased. But if you flip it 261 times and it comes up heads 200 times, you can be pretty sure something is going on.

Similarly, medical studies can be mathematically analyzed to determine whether their results are meaningful. There is more than one way to do this, and some methods have higher standards than others.

In the case of this study, one of the strictest mathematical techniques was used (technically, the U-test for study power). The results showed that these outcomes were extremely unlikely to have happened by chance.

The Mader study wasn't perfect, however. One problem was rather difficult to get around: garlic's odor. Twenty-one percent of study participants taking garlic had either noticed the odor themselves or heard others commenting on it. This gave them the clue that they were receiving the treatment rather than the placebo. In a double-blind study, as we've mentioned, participants are not supposed to know whether they're receiving the treatment or placebo. If 21% of the treatment group knew what they were receiving, this reduces the validity of the study. But it's not quite as bad as it sounds. Reportedly, 9% of the placebo group also claimed to smell a garlic odor on their bodies, which means that many people taking the placebo believed they were getting the treatment. Also, keep in mind that, in many double-blind studies of drugs, participants may be able to guess which group they are in based on the drug's side effects.[2]

Perhaps the most unfortunate aspect of this study was that it failed to evaluate garlic's effects on HDL and LDL cholesterol, which are actually more important than total cholesterol. Still, even with its flaws, this study gives us real evidence that garlic does reduce cholesterol levels.

What About HDL and LDL?

A study reported in 1993 did look at garlic's effects on HDL and LDL. It found positive results with LDL but no significant change in HDL. This double-blind placebo-controlled study enrolled 42 people whose total cholesterol levels were above 220 mg/dL.[3] Those in the treatment group took 300 mg of garlic powder (standardized to 1.3% alliin content) 3 times a day—slightly more than in the Mader study. Researchers measured total cholesterol, LDL cholesterol, HDL cholesterol, triglycerides, glucose (blood sugar), blood pressure, and heart rate during the 12-week study.

At the end of 12 weeks, the treatment group's total cholesterol had fallen from an average 262 mg/dL to 247 mg/dL, a 6% reduction. LDL ("bad") cholesterol decreased from 188 mg/dL to 168 mg/dL, an impressive 11% decrease. However, there was no significant change

Mary's Story

Mary was a 57-year-old woman who was reluctant to have her cholesterol level measured. "If it's high, I'll have to take drugs," she said. "I don't want to take drugs."

I explained that drugs weren't the only therapy—in fact, diet and exercise might be effective enough—but she said that she didn't want to exercise and found the idea of changing her diet "very depressing."

"You might try garlic," I said. "If your cholesterol's not too high."

The possibility of using a natural treatment gave Mary the courage to have her cholesterol checked. As it turned out, her total cholesterol level was only very slightly elevated, but it still needed to be reduced (it was 215). Her LDL also needed improvement, but her HDL was fine.

in the treatment group's HDL ("good") cholesterol levels. In the placebo group, none of these measures changed significantly.

While not a large study, this trial does suggest that garlic can improve LDL levels. However, more research is clearly needed.

Garlic Versus Conventional Medications

To date, only one study has been published comparing the efficacy of garlic to that of a conventional drug in reducing cholesterol and triglycerides. In 1992, a group of German researchers conducted a double-blind study comparing standardized garlic powder to bezafibrate (a drug prescribed in Germany).[4] Ninety-eight participants were en-

Even a mildly elevated cholesterol level is worth improving. We went over the available natural options, and she decided that of all the choices she'd prefer to try garlic. When we rechecked her lipid profile 2 months later, her total cholesterol and LDL cholesterol levels had gone back to normal.

Mary's cholesterol was only a little bit high, within the range that garlic might be able to help. What would I have done if her cholesterol level had been more significantly elevated? Given her preferences, I probably would have suggested she try other natural supplements that appear to be more effective than garlic, such as policosanol and stanols (see chapter 4). If those steps were not successful, I would have presented her with the choice of making the lifestyle changes she wanted to avoid or using medications in the statin family.

—Steven Bratman, M.D.

rolled and randomly assigned to receive either garlic or bezafibrate. The results over 12 weeks showed that 900 mg of standardized garlic powder daily was equally effective to 600 mg of bezafibrate. Both reduced total cholesterol by about 25%.

However, there's one problem with this study: both groups of participants made important dietary changes. This may have tended to hide real differences in treatment outcome.

Aged Garlic: May Also Be Effective

Nearly all the studies that have found garlic effective at reducing cholesterol used powdered garlic standardized to its alliin content. However, several studies used garlic that was simply aged, without any attempt to keep alliin intact. Because its processing is simpler, aged garlic is relatively inexpensive. There is some evidence that aged garlic may also lower cholesterol, but it may not lower it to the same extent as garlic processed to preserve the alliin.

In one study, 41 men with moderately high cholesterol took either placebo or 7.2 g of aged garlic extract daily for 4 to 6 months.[5] Aged garlic reduced total cholesterol by 6.1% more than placebo and reduced LDL by 4.6% more than placebo.

While positive, these results were less impressive than what has been seen in studies of garlic powder standardized to 1.3% alliin. However, since there have not been any head-to-head comparisons, we can't really say for sure that aged garlic is less effective than standardized powdered garlic. Nonetheless, many experts suspect that it is weaker, because it contains fewer of the probable active ingredients.

On the Other Hand: Studies That Found Standardized Garlic Powder Ineffective

Four recent studies using standardized garlic powder did not come up with positive results.

In the first study, a total of 115 individuals were followed for 6 months.[6] Half received 900 mg of dried garlic powder daily (standardized to 1.3% allicin) and the other half received a matching placebo that was coated with garlic powder (too little to produce any therapeutic effect) so it would be indistinguishable from the actual garlic tablet. The surprising results showed no benefits in any measured factors, including total cholesterol, triglycerides, LDL, or HDL levels.

Three other studies have also found garlic ineffective.[7,8,9]

What is the explanation for this discrepancy? A close look shows that, in the four negative studies, all participants were put on a lowfat diet—a standard procedure when studying conventional cholesterol-lowering medications. In addition, some natural treatments such as policosanol and red yeast rice have proven effective in such studies. However, garlic is not a tremendously effective cholesterol-reducing agent; putting everyone on a low-cholesterol diet seems to overwhelm the effects of the herb.

Another potential explanation may lie in the nature of the garlic used. Reportedly, many of the most commonly used garlic powder supplements manufactured from 1995 to 1997 were of relatively poor quality.[10]

The Bottom Line

Putting together all the evidence on garlic for high cholesterol, it appears that the herb does offer some benefit overall. However, the effect is relatively modest.[11]

How Does Garlic Reduce Cholesterol?

The exact mechanism by which garlic lowers cholesterol is not really clear, although we have some intriguing clues. While no one chemical in garlic has been shown to be the single active ingredient, most researchers would probably agree that the sulfur-containing compounds are responsible for the cholesterol-lowering effect. Let's take a closer look.

As described previously, garlic contains a chemical called alliin. Most of the studies described earlier used a form of garlic in which alliin is carefully preserved. Once in the body, the alliin breaks down into allicin and other substances including ajoene, vinyldithiins, diallyl disulfide, and diallyl trisulfide (see figure 4). These substances are rapidly absorbed.[12] These garlic constituents then apparently help decrease the production of cholesterol by blocking an enzyme known as HMG-CoA reductase.[13] (Statin drugs work

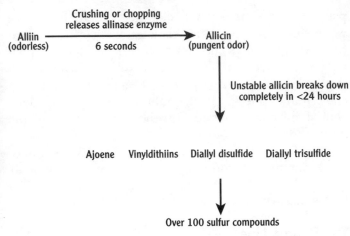

Figure 4. *Breakdown of garlic's sulfur-containing compounds*

in a similar manner. We'll discuss them in more detail in chapter 7.) We don't know precisely which of these garlic components are most important, however. Allicin may be one of the most significant,[14,15] but other constituents appear to play a role as well.[16–19]

The upshot of all these studies appears to be that garlic produces its effects on cholesterol in more than one way, and its various constituents may work together to produce a combined effect. However, there is still much we do not know.

Beyond Cholesterol: Other Heart-Healthy Benefits of Garlic

Garlic's effect on cholesterol isn't its only benefit for treating and preventing atherosclerosis. Several double-blind studies suggest that garlic modestly, but meaningfully, reduces blood pressure, which is a known risk factor for atherosclerosis. The combined benefits of reducing both cholesterol and blood pressure make garlic a promising all-around preventive treatment for atherosclerosis. Not only that, other studies suggest that garlic's usefulness in treating and preventing atherosclerosis goes beyond its effects on either cholesterol or blood pressure. So we have to look further. Some possibilities for other positive effects include garlic's known ability to "thin" the blood and fight free radicals.

Several double-blind studies suggest that garlic modestly, but meaningfully, reduces blood pressure, which is a known risk factor for atherosclerosis.

In this section, we'll explore all the other ways garlic may protect your arteries. We'll also present evidence from an exciting study, which suggests that regular use of garlic can reduce the risk of heart attacks.

Garlic and High Blood Pressure

There is some evidence that garlic can reduce high blood pressure (or *hypertension*), at least modestly. Part of this evidence comes from animal studies.[20,21] Additionally, in studies evaluating garlic's effects on cholesterol, researchers have noticed reductions in blood pressure as a kind of positive "side effect." Finally, a few human studies have focused directly on garlic's effect on blood pressure as their primary interest. The overall results suggest that garlic can indeed meaningfully reduce blood pressure.

One of the studies of garlic's effects on high blood pressure was a 1990 double-blind placebo-controlled study of 47 individuals.[22] This 12-week trial enrolled people with mild hypertension. Participants were given either 600 mg of garlic powder or a similar-looking placebo.

At the end of the study, the group given garlic showed a significant reduction in blood pressure. The diastolic blood pressure (the bottom number in blood pressure readings) had fallen by about 11 mm Hg (millimeters of mercury), whereas those taking placebo had no significant change.

Systolic blood pressure (the top number of the blood pressure reading) also fell considerably in the group taking the garlic. There was a 20 mm Hg average drop in the garlic group versus no significant change in the placebo group.

In other words, participants who began with a reading of 170/100 ended up with a much closer to normal blood pressure of 150/89. (See figures 5 and 6). Although the systolic blood pressure reading was still too high, blood pressure was much better overall. There were no reports of side effects, and only three participants mentioned that they noticed a slight garlic odor.

However, this study suffered from a significant flaw: The average blood pressure in the garlic-treated group was 171/102, while in the placebo group it was 161/97. This difference is somewhat larger than it should be. The two groups in a double-blind study should start out as virtually identical on average in order to avoid comparing apples and oranges.

Positive results have been seen in other studies as well, although they too were flawed. In 1994, Professor Christopher Silagy and Dr. Andrew Neil from Oxford University conducted a review of all the human studies published at that time on garlic's influence on blood pressure.[23] To be included in their review, each study had to use a double-blind design, last at least 4 weeks, and satisfy other requirements to ensure that the results were

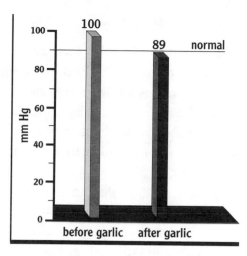

Figure 5. *Example of reduction in diastolic blood pressure in treatment (garlic) group after 12 weeks in a double-blind study* (Auer, 1990)

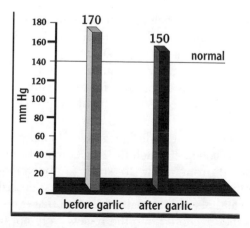

Figure 6. *Example of reduction in systolic blood pressure in treatment (garlic) group after 12 weeks in a double-blind study* (Auer, 1990)

Patty's Story

Patty, 52, went to see Dr. Robin Dipasquale for help in improving her overall health. Patty had many health concerns, but she was primarily anxious about her high blood pressure. She was already taking conventional drugs to control her blood pressure, but it was still high at 172/104 mm Hg, and she wanted Dr. Dipasquale to help her bring it down further.

Patty was extremely afraid that she would have a heart attack, and she was upset that her current medications were not as successful as she had hoped they would be. Dr. Dipasquale recommended standard dietary and lifestyle changes and started Patty on 900 mg per day of a garlic extract standardized to contain 1.3% alliin. Patty was to continue her regular medications as well and return in 1 month.

meaningful. Eight trials met these requirements. They all used dried garlic powder standardized to 1.3% alliin in doses ranging from 600 to 900 mg per day. The average duration of the trials was about 12 weeks, and a total of 415 subjects were involved. However, only three of the studies involved people with high blood pressure.

When pooled together, the overall results of these studies suggest that garlic can reduce blood pressure better than placebo, although the exact amount of the reduction varied from study to study. Improvements were similar to those seen in the 1990 study just described.

The authors of this analysis caution that even the eight studies they accepted into the review were not top-notch; like the one described previously, they all suffered from a number of scientific imperfections. We really need larger, longer, and better-designed studies. Nonetheless, the

When Patty came back, her blood pressure had decreased dramatically, by almost 25%. Over the course of the next year, Patty stayed on the garlic extract, and she was able to cut back on her blood pressure medication considerably. At her last follow-up, her blood pressure was stable at 138/76.

In Patty's case, it is not clear whether it was the lifestyle changes or the garlic that had the most impact. Nonetheless, physicians frequently combine drugs that individually reduce high blood pressure in hopes of achieving a greater effect than with any single one alone; it certainly makes sense to use garlic in the same way.

Warning: Because we don't know how garlic interacts with other medications, we recommend physician supervision when combining the herb with blood pressure drugs.

available evidence does suggest that garlic can meaningfully reduce blood pressure. The researchers point out that this effect, if sustained over a long period of time, could add up to a major health benefit, reducing strokes by 30 to 40% and heart disease by 20 to 25%.

Although there are several theories that try to explain how garlic might work to reduce blood pressure, we don't really know for sure which one is correct. Our best guess is that garlic dilates blood vessels. When the vessels become wider, more blood can flow through with less resistance, reducing blood pressure.

But how does garlic dilate blood vessels? One theory suggests that garlic relaxes the artery walls by stimulating the production of nitric oxide.[24,25] Nitric oxide is a natural substance that the body itself releases to relax the muscles that line arteries. However, this theory is far from proven.[26]

Another theory suggests that garlic may work like a family of blood pressure medications known as calcium channel–blockers. These drugs relax the artery wall by blocking the entrance of calcium into cells, thereby causing them to relax (for reasons that are too complex to delve into here). Several laboratory studies have found that both garlic and its individual constituents can affect the way calcium moves into smooth muscle cells.[27,28] However, as yet, there have been no human studies showing the same effect.

The bottom line is that while garlic does appear to reduce blood pressure, we don't know exactly how it works.

Other Effects on Atherosclerosis

Given that garlic can reduce cholesterol and blood pressure, one would certainly expect it to reduce the rate of atherosclerosis. Animal studies definitely indicate that this is the case. According to a review published in 1997, at least 16 controlled animal studies have been performed evaluating garlic's effects on atherosclerosis.[29] Twelve of the studies found that garlic protects against the formation of atherosclerosis. Furthermore, three studies found that it can actually reverse atherosclerosis. Only one study did not find any benefit.

While these results are exciting, you have to keep in mind that there was a certain artificiality to all of them. These were not laboratory animals that just happened to develop atherosclerosis; rather, researchers stimulated it by one artificial means or another. In some studies, an artery wall was deliberately damaged, while in others, animals were fed a diet designed to dramatically speed atherosclerosis. Still, these findings are definitely promising, and they deserve to be taken seriously.

It's much harder to study atherosclerosis in people. Not only would it be unethical to deliberately give people atherosclerosis, most methods used to measure the extent of mild atherosclerosis are dangerous or at least unpleasant.

However, one study used a very clever approach to discover whether garlic reduces atherosclerosis in people. This study, published in 1997, estimated the extent of atherosclerosis by looking at the elasticity of the largest artery in the body, the aorta.[30] As atherosclerosis advances, the aorta becomes stiffer. In general, the older you are, the stiffer the aorta becomes because just about everyone develops some atherosclerosis over time. There is a special (and extremely technical) technique known as *pulse wave velocity measurement* that can evaluate the elasticity of the aorta without posing any risk to the participant.

The study followed 101 matched pairs of people between ages 50 and 80, who were carefully selected to be similar in every important way except for their use of garlic. One group consisted of those who reported taking more than 300 mg of standardized garlic powder per day for at least 2 years. The other group was similar in age, sex, and weight but did not take garlic on a regular basis.

These two groups were then evaluated using the pulse wave velocity measurement technique. The results were positive and unmistakable: Individuals who used garlic regularly had much more flexible aortas. Thus, regular garlic use was associated with less atherosclerosis. These results strongly suggest that garlic use can slow down the development of atherosclerosis.

This study had one surprising feature: People taking garlic developed less atherosclerosis even though their cholesterol level and blood pressure were identical (on average) to those who did not take it. This suggests that garlic's atherosclerosis-fighting powers are greater than the sum of its effects on cholesterol and blood pressure. Some other action or actions must be at work as well.

Garlic and Blood Clotting

Garlic's "blood-thinning" effects may be part of the explanation for its ability to treat and prevent atherosclerosis. Garlic appears to both help prevent blood clots from forming and help break down clots that have already developed. As we saw in chapter 1, blood clots play a role in atherosclerosis. These clots not only add to the layer of plaque coating blood vessel walls, they can also break loose and become lodged further down the bloodstream, causing a stroke or heart attack.

One commonly prescribed preventive treatment for heart disease is taking one baby aspirin a day. Aspirin is a blood thinner, which is believed to be at least one reason why it helps. It works by interfering with platelets, cells that start the formation of a clot. Platelets (as you may recall from chapter 1) normally circulate throughout our arteries and veins, waiting to repair any leaks. When they find an injured or leaking artery, they attach to it, quickly forming a plug.

Garlic's "blood-thinning" effects may be part of the explanation for its ability to treat and prevent atherosclerosis.

Unfortunately, platelets see atherosclerosis as "injury" to our bodies, and act as if the plaque was a bleeding artery. The platelets surround the plaque and begin to stick to both the lesion and each other. This sets off a cascade of events which, as we've seen, can lead to a disaster for your health. Chemicals released by platelets may also accelerate atherosclerosis.

Like aspirin, one of the ways garlic intervenes in clot formation is by keeping the platelets from sticking to each other. If the platelets can't clump easily, then a clot is less likely to form. Several studies have found that garlic and its constituents can reduce the ability of platelets to adhere to each other and to plaque.[31–35]

Warning: If you have been advised to take aspirin to help prevent heart attacks, we do not recommend substituting garlic for it except on the advice of a physician. We don't know if garlic is as effective as aspirin for this purpose.

Garlic has another effect besides helping prevent clots from forming. It seems to help break down existing blood clots. It does so by dissolving a protein called *fibrin,* which is the "webbing" of a clot.[36] This dissolving action is called *fibrinolysis.* Clot-dissolving drugs are used in the immediate stages after a heart attack or stroke.

Garlic appears to both help prevent blood clots from forming and help break down clots that have already developed.

The drugs used to break down clots immediately after heart attacks are much more potent—too potent to be taken long term. Garlic's effect certainly doesn't seem to be strong enough to make garlic a good alternative to drugs in emergencies. But perhaps garlic will prove to be effective enough to be used as a preventive measure in treating blood clots. At this point, we don't have the answer. Interestingly, even cooked garlic seems to dissolve clots to some extent.[37]

Another Possibility: Garlic As an Antioxidant

One theory suggests that free radicals are an important cause of atherosclerosis. Free radicals are naturally occurring molecules that can damage many of our tissues. They can also attack LDL ("bad") cholesterol and make it even more harmful to arteries.

Can Garlic's "Blood-Thinning" Effects Be Dangerous?

We've said that garlic decreases blood clotting, but what does that really mean? Well, you don't necessarily need to worry about bleeding to death if you cut yourself while taking garlic. Garlic is definitely not this powerful! However, garlic's influence on blood clotting does suggest that it might be risky to combine it with blood-thinning drugs, or perhaps even natural supplements that also thin the blood. It also might not be a good idea to take garlic immediately before or after surgery or labor and delivery, and people with blood clotting disorders should definitely seek medical advice.

A number of substances called *antioxidants* help the body combat the damaging effects of oxidation. Garlic is a potent antioxidant, and it appears to protect LDL cholesterol from free radicals.[38–41] Several studies have identified some of garlic's sulfur compounds as antioxidants, including alliin and allicin as well as two other compounds called S-allyl cysteine and diallyl disulfide.[42,43] Other studies on garlic indicate that it is also an effective neutralizer of free radicals.[44,45]

The Bottom Line: Does Garlic Reduce Deaths from Heart Disease?

The study we discussed previously, which measured the elasticity of the aorta to see if garlic could reduce atherosclerosis, is not the only one that has found general benefits against atherosclerosis. In a double-blind placebo-controlled study that followed 152 individuals for 4 years, standardized garlic powder at a dosage of 900 mg daily significantly slowed the development of atherosclerosis as measured by ultrasound.[46] Although this study suffered from some statistical flaws, it nonetheless provides additional direct evidence that all of garlic's effects combine to protect against hardening of the arteries. And if your arteries don't harden, you probably won't have a heart attack.

A controlled study published in 1989 provides direct evidence that garlic prevents heart attacks and heart attack death. This 3-year study followed 432 individuals who had previously suffered a heart attack.[47] Half of the participants received garlic oil equivalent to about 2 g daily of fresh garlic, while the others did not receive any treatment. All participants continued to take whatever standard medications they had been prescribed.

The results were very impressive. Those who had taken the garlic had a significant reduction in both mortality from heart attacks (45%) and in the recurrence of heart attacks (35%). This finding is in many ways the most significant one we've discussed so far. Although the study is not perfect (it didn't use a placebo treatment), the results nonetheless suggest that garlic's effects are not just theoretically beneficial, but that they actually add up to longer life and fewer heart attacks.

Dosage

Now that you have read about the benefits of garlic, you may be ready to start taking it.

The best-studied form of garlic is a garlic powder preparation standardized to contain 1.3% alliin. The usual dose of this type of garlic is 300 mg taken 2 to 3 times daily. Check the label to make sure it says "provides 10 mg

Options for Enjoying Fresh Garlic

If you decide to try fresh, whole garlic, there are some delicious alternatives to simply chewing up a clove at a time. Try eating it on your salad in a freshly made garlic dressing: Crush 1 or more cloves of garlic (a garlic press is a handy tool) and add olive oil and balsamic vinegar to taste. Experiment with different vinegars and seasonings such as oregano, basil, pepper, and mustard. (Keep in mind that if you put this dressing in the refrigerator, you are making aged garlic.)

If you like Middle Eastern food, you can make hummus: Blend some cooked, cooled garbanzo beans together and add small amounts, to taste, of tahini (sesame paste), olive oil, lemon juice, salt (if your blood pressure allows), and fresh garlic. Use it as a dip for vegetables, or spread it on pita bread.

(or 10,000 mcg) alliin daily" or "4 mg (4,000 mcg) allicin potential daily."

These statements refer to the fact, mentioned earlier, that garlic contains a substance called alliin, which in turn becomes the presumed active ingredient allicin. Because allicin itself is unstable, many manufacturers attempt to provide a set amount of alliin instead. The alliin then turns to allicin in your body when you consume it.

Aged garlic, on the other hand, contains no alliin, and therefore does not release allicin in the body. Some Japanese researchers have argued that allicin is harmful and that aged garlic is safer. While other authorities do not agree, most of the safety studies we describe in the following section have used aged garlic, and it is probably the one form that we know for sure is completely safe. Nonetheless, the use of aged garlic remains controversial. Be-

Hard-core garlic lovers will eat it raw in just about anything: pizza (sprinkle chopped, fresh garlic on a cooked pizza the minute it leaves the oven), soups and stews (use a garlic press to add fresh garlic just before serving), or even blended up in a vegetable-juice smoothie.

Of course, cooked garlic is found in many foods. Unfortunately, it probably isn't effective for reducing cholesterol. It does not contain the same amount of active ingredients as freshly cut, raw garlic, so baking, roasting, sautéing, or frying your medicinal garlic most likely will not give you the same cholesterol-lowering benefit. However, evidence suggests that garlic in food may help prevent cancer, particularly cancer of the colon and stomach.[48–55] So it's still worth it!

cause it lacks alliin, allicin, and other constituents that are believed to be medically active in reducing cholesterol and heart disease, many authorities feel that it is distinctly inferior. However, two things can be said for it: Aged garlic is nearly odor-free, and it is very easy on the stomach. The typical dose is 1 to 7.2 g daily.

Fresh garlic may be the strongest form of garlic available (at least theoretically). By definition, all of the therapeutic ingredients are present in garlic cloves. These ingredients are released during chewing. A typical dose is 1 or 2 cloves daily. While this is certainly a cheap, easy way to take garlic, it has some serious problems—primarily the taste and smell. Cooked garlic, however, is probably not effective.

Finally, garlic oil products are available. Garlic oil does not appear to reduce cholesterol levels. However, it does seem to have some heart-healthy benefits, and it was a form of garlic that prevented death from heart attacks in the large 3-year study described earlier.

Side Effects and Safety Issues

Garlic appears to be a relatively safe herb. The most serious concerns, as we'll describe in this section, have to do with possible risks of bleeding. However, the biggest problem with garlic is not a typical side effect at all: odor.

Garlic Breath

Garlic's most commonly reported side effect is annoying rather than dangerous: the smell. Even "odorless" garlic products produce this problem to some extent. Although it is not significant in terms of health, as many as 30% of those who try garlic give it up for this reason.

One double-blind study set out to specifically investigate garlic breath.[56] The study looked at the effects of

> **Garlic's most commonly reported side effect is annoying rather than dangerous: odor.**

daily doses of 300 mg, 600 mg, 900 mg, or 1,200 mg of standardized garlic powder. Participants were asked to keep an odor log and record if and when they noticed a garlic smell on their breath or in their sweat.

As you might expect, higher doses of garlic caused people to notice more garlic odor. Daily doses of 900 to 1,200 mg were associated with a 50% incidence of noticeable fragrance. The authors note that this effect frequently prompts individuals to reduce their dose and speculate that participants enrolled in studies may have done so as well, potentially reducing garlic's apparent effectiveness.

However, not everyone dislikes the smell of garlic, and different individuals experience different degrees of odor. People who have trouble with garlic odor might try switching to another kind of garlic product before giving up on it as an herbal medicine.

"Odorless" garlic powder products are not truly odorless, but they do cause little to no immediate garlic breath. The reason is that they don't release allicin until they proceed for awhile down the intestinal tract. However, once it is produced, allicin travels through the body and causes odor to arise from the lungs or skin.

Thus, while these products are much less smelly than garlic itself, they don't fully eliminate this side effect. Aged garlic may be even better, because it doesn't produce any allicin at all.

> **People who have trouble with garlic odor might try switching to another kind of garlic product before giving it up altogether.**

Other Side Effects

Participants in garlic studies have reported a few other minor side effects besides odor. However, these are probably not actual problems caused by garlic. The reason we say this is that in the double-blind placebo-controlled studies of garlic, the incidence of side effects aside from odor was never any higher than what was seen in the placebo group.

Yes, people taking placebo report side effects! It's not uncommon for as many as 20 to 30% of people given placebo treatments to report such problems as headaches, nausea, fatigue, dizziness, and allergic reactions. Just as taking a pill can make you feel better through the power of suggestion, it seems that just the idea of taking a pill is enough to make some people feel sick.

In one study of 261 individuals, fewer than 1% of those taking garlic reported minor stomach upset, while about 2.5% of those taking placebo experienced the same problem.[57] It is most likely that the stomachaches seen in the garlic group were not truly caused by the garlic, any more than the side effects in the placebo group were caused by placebo.

A large study performed in 1993 evaluated 1,997 individuals to see if taking 900 mg of garlic daily would cause any serious side effects.[58] Studies of this type are called "drug monitoring" studies. They don't involve a placebo group, but simply follow a large group of people for an extended period of time, looking for rare or delayed problems. This study lasted 16 weeks.

Researchers asked study participants about their experiences with side effects at the beginning of the study and again after 8 and 16 weeks of treatment. No serious side effects were observed. The most common complaint was nausea (6%), followed by dizziness on standing up (1.3%), and allergic reaction to garlic (1.1%). Less than 1% reported other complaints such as bloating, headaches, dizziness at rest, and sweating. However, since there was no placebo group in this study, it can't be determined what proportion of these side effects were real. The major evidence provided by this study is that garlic causes no dangerous side effects.

However, raw garlic appears to be able to cause more side effects than the garlic preparations usually used in studies. Symptoms such as heartburn, upset stomach, headache, flushed skin, rapid pulse, insomnia, flatulence, and diarrhea have all been reported by people who ate large amounts of fresh garlic. Some people are particularly intolerant of garlic, and they experience some gastrointestinal complaints even when they eat just a little.

In addition, there have been several reports of fresh garlic causing contact *dermatitis* (a rash on the skin).[59,60,61] As the name implies, this is an allergic condition that appears after touching garlic. It usually manifests as a red, often scaly rash wherever the garlic touched, such as the palms of the hands. Most of these cases were in people who handled a lot of raw garlic on a regular basis: caterers, cooks, farmers, and homemakers. There are no reports that handling other garlic preparations can cause this problem.

Toxicity

Toxicity is a slightly different issue from side effects. This term usually refers to a substance's ability to cause severe harm when taken in excessive doses. Many substances can be toxic if you take enough. But some are more toxic than others.

Scientists measure toxicity by determining how large a dose is required to kill 50% of a given group of laboratory animals. This dose is called the LD_{50}, meaning the lethal dose in 50%.

We know much more about the safety of aged garlic than other forms of garlic. In one study, rats were given up to 2,000 mg of aged garlic extract per kilogram body weight for a period of 6 months.[62] No toxic symptoms were observed, and examination of organs and tissue found no hidden damage. The only thing that researchers noticed was that rats that were given garlic ate less than the control group. (Maybe garlic should be marketed as a diet aid!)

To put this dose in perspective, consider that the amount given to the rats is equivalent to about 120 to 150 g per day for an average-sized person. Since the recommended dose of aged garlic is 1 to 7.2 g daily, you will see that there is a large margin of safety.

Henry's Story

Henry, age 54, had a persistent problem with mildly elevated cholesterol (230 mg/dL), despite his best efforts at improving his lifestyle. His LDL ("bad") cholesterol was somewhat elevated as well, and his HDL ("good") level was just barely adequate.

Unfortunately, none of the treatments he had tried to improve his cholesterol level had worked out. Every one of them had irritated his liver. Two different statin drugs, the fibric acid derivative clofibrate, and the vitamin supplement niacin (see chapter 3 for more information on niacin) had all caused his liver enzymes to rise (a sign of liver irritation and/or damage).

However, aged garlic is known to contain virtually no alliin, allicin, or disulfides. It may be that other forms of garlic, such as raw garlic or garlic standardized to alliin, are more toxic. Since there have been no animal toxicity studies on garlic powder standardized to alliin content, we don't really know for sure. This is unfortunate because nearly all the clinical trials used this type of garlic powder.

Aged garlic has also been tested for *genotoxicity* (damage to the genetic material) and *mutagenicity* (ability to cause mutations in the genetic material).[63] The results suggest that garlic doesn't increase the risk of cancer—at least not by damaging or causing mutations in the genes. Unfortunately, once more, there have been no comparable studies of standardized garlic powder.

Garlic and the Blood

One potential risk of garlic definitely deserves mention. As mentioned earlier, garlic interferes with platelets (which

His doctor suggested that the hepatitis he had had as a child might have left his liver hypersensitive. But this left Henry in a quandary. He didn't want to ignore his high cholesterol levels. However, since he already exercised for 60 minutes daily and ate as little fat as he could, he didn't know what else to do.

Another doctor suggested that he try taking standardized garlic powder at a dose of 900 mg daily. Within 1 month, his total cholesterol had fallen to 205 mg/dL, and, based on his LDL and HDL levels, this was a sufficient reduction. Best of all, his liver enzymes remained normal.

are responsible for blood clotting) and may also help the body to dissolve existing blood clots. This may mean that garlic can cause excessive bleeding in certain individuals.

In 1990, there was a case report of *spontaneous spinal epidural hematoma* (spontaneous bleeding around the spinal cord) occurring in an 87-year-old man who claimed to be eating 4 cloves of raw garlic daily. It's not clear whether the garlic really had anything to do with his condition, because in 41% of individuals with this condition, no cause is ever determined. Still, to be on the safe side, certain people should consult a physician before using garlic. In particular, we would certainly recommend caution if you have a bleeding disorder (such as hemophilia). Furthermore, if you are about to have surgery, have just had surgery, or are pregnant and nearly ready to deliver, garlic might not be a good idea.

Surgery and childbirth inevitably involve bleeding, and there has been one report of increased bleeding following

TURP surgery (the primary treatment for enlarged prostate gland) in a man who took garlic.[64] Another report described excessive bleeding in a woman undergoing breast surgery.[65] Because you want your blood to clot normally and stop the bleeding, you should avoid taking garlic supplements for 2 weeks or so before surgery or childbirth and during the recovery period. As we'll see in the next section, an even greater concern involves potential interactions between garlic and blood-thinning medications.

Drug Interactions

There are serious concerns that garlic might interact with blood-thinning medications. Some of these medications, such as Coumadin, are rather touchy drugs, and various medications (and even foods) can affect their action. It is very possible that garlic's slight blood-thinning effect could combine with the more powerful effect of such medications and lead to *excessive* thinning of the blood. The results could be dangerous, especially if you were to get in an automobile accident while taking both at once.

The most powerful drugs in this category are warfarin (Coumadin) and heparin. Aspirin and Trental (pentoxifylline) also interfere with blood clotting to a much more modest extent. If you are taking any medications of this type, you should consult your physician before taking garlic. Furthermore, a few natural substances are also mild blood thinners, such as the herb ginkgo, the supplement policosanol, and vitamin E. Conceivably, bleeding problems might develop when you combine these treatments, although no such problems have been reported.

Garlic may also combine poorly with certain HIV medications. Two people with HIV experienced severe gastrointestinal symptoms when taking the HIV drug ritonavir and garlic supplements.[66]

Garlic in Specific Medical Circumstances

Based on indirect evidence, people in certain medical circumstances might want to be especially cautious in using garlic.

Pemphigus

Pemphigus is a rare autoimmune disease that involves the skin and mucous membranes. Characterized by large, fluid-filled blisters and thickening of the skin, it most often occurs in people between 30 and 60 years of age, and it can be fatal.

A certain chemical compound called a *thiol group* can worsen pemphigus. Since garlic contains an active thiol group, there are some concerns that it might potentially cause a similar problem. For the same reason, people with this disease are cautioned to avoid other foods in the garlic family such as leeks, onions, shallots, and chives.

> **It is very possible that garlic's slight blood-thinning effect could combine with the more powerful effect of medications such as Coumadin and lead to bleeding problems.**

Organ Transplants

At high doses, garlic has been shown to activate certain cells of the immune system called natural killer (NK) cells.[67,68] These are a type of white blood cell that patrols our bodies looking for bacteria, viruses, and other invaders and helps to remove them. People who receive organ transplants don't want their natural killer cells activated, because these cells can cause organ transplant rejection. NK cells may attack the new organ as if it were an enemy. Organ transplant recipients are usually treated with drugs that suppress NK cells—as well as other parts of the immune system—to keep the transplanted organ safe. Garlic could conceivably reverse this suppression.

Diabetes

Weak evidence suggests that garlic may lower blood sugar (glucose). If true, this could make it paradoxically both helpful and dangerous for people with diabetes. The danger would come if garlic caused a sudden or unanticipated drop in blood sugar levels (hypoglycemia). People with diabetes are often skirting the edge of hypoglycemia, and a sudden drop in blood sugar can be dangerous. On the other hand, if garlic has a mild, gentle effect of reducing blood sugar, it could conceivably play a helpful role in maintaining a healthy blood sugar level.

However, there's not much evidence to suggest that garlic actually reduces blood sugar levels. Some animal studies have found this effect, while others have not, and it has not been seen in human studies. Still, to be on the safe side, if you have diabetes and are considering whether or not to use garlic, consult your physician to assess the potential risk of altering your blood sugar levels.

Long-Term Risks

A question people often ask about herbs is whether it is safe to take them for many years. This is a legitimate concern because many drugs cause problems that only become evident after a long period of use, and herbs could conceivably do the same thing.

There is some evidence that long-term consumption of garlic as a food actually reduces the risk of cancer.[69] However, since most people eat cooked garlic, which is very different from typical garlic supplements, these findings really say little about the safety of long-term use of garlic powder.

Some people feel that because garlic is a natural herb, it is more likely than a drug to be safe in the long run. However, this is more of an emotional statement than a rational one. Numerous herbs have been shown to be potentially toxic, including comfrey and chaparral. For that matter, fatty foods appear to be carcinogenic. In other words, there is no guarantee that garlic is completely safe just because it's natural. We simply don't know.

There is no guarantee that garlic is completely safe just because it's natural.

What About Pregnant or Nursing Women?

There haven't been any animal or human studies that specifically examined whether standardized garlic powder affects embryos, fetuses, or young children. Therefore, safety cannot be assured for pregnant or nursing women.

Finally, as mentioned previously, garlic probably shouldn't be used in the weeks prior to labor and delivery.

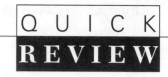

- Garlic has been used as both a food and medicine by cultures worldwide for more than 5,000 years.

- We do not know for certain what the active ingredient is in garlic, but it is believed to be a substance called allicin. Many (but not all) manufacturers of garlic powder for medicinal use attempt to provide a set amount of alliin (a related substance that spontaneously turns into allicin).

- Garlic appears to modestly reduce cholesterol levels.

- Garlic may also lower elevated blood pressure.

- Garlic may prevent blood platelets from sticking together and increase the body's ability to break down blood clots.

- Garlic is a potent antioxidant. Antioxidants may help prevent atherosclerosis by protecting LDL ("bad") cholesterol from being turned into an even more dangerous form.

- Putting all these effects together, garlic appears to help prevent atherosclerosis and reduce death from heart disease. However, more research is needed.

- The proper dose of garlic will depend on the form you are taking. The most common dose is 300 mg 2 to 3 times daily of garlic powder standardized to contain 1.3% alliin. This will provide a daily dose of about 10 mg (10,000 mcg) of alliin daily, or a total allicin potential of 4 mg (4,000 mcg) daily.

- Garlic appears to be a relatively safe herb with very few side effects. The most frequent problem is odor. If this problem occurs with a garlic product (as opposed to fresh garlic) it might be fixed by trying a different brand.

- Garlic should be avoided by people with pemphigus, hard to control diabetes, or those who are just about to—or who have just undergone—surgery or labor and delivery. Individuals taking blood pressure–lowering drugs or medications for HIV should also not use garlic.

- There are some concerns that garlic may cause bleeding problems if combined with blood-thinning medications, or with other natural supplements that thin the blood.

- Garlic's safety for pregnant or nursing mothers has not been established.

Niacin and High Cholesterol

N iacin is a water-soluble vitamin, also known as vitamin B_3, that serves many functions in our bodies. It interacts with more than 200 enzymes that help our bodies metabolize fats and sugars and produce energy. Niacin can be found in most animal products, such as liver and other organ meats, poultry, and fish, but it is also found in many plant sources like sesame and sunflower seeds, whole grains, red chili peppers, nuts (especially peanuts, almonds, and pine nuts), and avocados.

Technically, niacin is a nonessential vitamin, meaning that we can live without getting it in our diet. Our bodies are able to make it from another common nutrient, the amino acid *tryptophan,* along with the help of vitamins B_1, B_2, B_6, and C, as well as iron. Nonetheless, most people get plenty of already-formed niacin from the foods they eat, and there is an official minimum daily recommendation that will "cover" your niacin needs even if other nutrients are missing (see sidebar, Niacin: Diet Versus Supplements).

Niacin: Diet Versus Supplements

Many foods provide high amounts of niacin. The best sources include brewer's yeast; rice bran; wheat bran; peanuts; organ meats, such as liver; and certain types of fish, such as trout, halibut, swordfish, and salmon. Other good sources of niacin are whole grains, wheat germ, pine nuts, sunflower seeds, and split peas.

The U.S. recommendation for daily intake of niacin for an adult is between 14 and 16 mg daily. Since many foods provide between 7 and 38 mg per 3.5-ounce portion of the food, meeting the dietary requirement typically is not a problem.

Niacin can also lower cholesterol. When used for this purpose, it must be taken in amounts much higher than what is manufactured by the body or found in food. This use of niacin was discovered many decades ago, and at one time niacin was the most commonly used conventional treatment for high cholesterol.

The U.S. National Cholesterol Education Program (NCEP) considers niacin to be in the same league as the lipid-lowering drugs discussed in chapter 7. NCEP further suggests that niacin is especially valuable in treating high cholesterol in individuals with low HDL cholesterol, and in those with both high cholesterol and high triglycerides.

Since the advent of the statin drugs, however, most physicians have stopped using niacin. This is due in part to the fact that the statin drugs have shown to be more effective in reducing both total cholesterol and LDL ("bad") cholesterol levels. Niacin has also been associated with annoying (as well as potentially dangerous) side effects. Nevertheless, it is still a highly effective treatment for high

However, it is unlikely that you could achieve high enough doses in your diet to get the therapeutic effect. For example, peanuts contain about 16 mg of niacin per 3.5-ounce portion. If you consider that the dose of niacin required to lower cholesterol is about 1,500 mg daily, then you would have to eat almost 328 ounces of peanuts each day, which is about 20 pounds of peanuts! It is doubtful most people would be able to eat 140 pounds of peanuts each week (not to mention afford buying such large quantities). You really have to take niacin supplements if you wish to use it to improve your cholesterol levels.

cholesterol that is safe if used properly. Not only can niacin improve cholesterol levels, it has also been shown to improve overall mortality.[1] Additionally, niacin is one of the few treatments that can dramatically improve HDL ("good") cholesterol levels.

What Is the Scientific Evidence for Niacin?

There is very strong scientific evidence supporting the use of niacin. We will not go into it in

Niacin is a highly effective treatment for high cholesterol, and it is safe if used properly.

great detail, because niacin's effectiveness is not in question. Unlike garlic, it is used in conventional medicine, and niacin has been approved by the FDA.

Several well-designed double-blind placebo-controlled studies have found that niacin reduced LDL cholesterol by approximately 10%, decreased triglycerides by 25%, and raised HDL cholesterol by 20 to 30%.[2–8] Niacin also lowers levels of lipoprotein(a)—another risk factor for atherosclerosis—by about 35%.

Other studies have compared niacin with statin drugs, the most effective and widely used conventional treatments for high cholesterol. These studies have consistently shown that the statin drugs are more effective than niacin when it comes to reducing total cholesterol and LDL cholesterol, but that niacin is more effective in lowering triglycerides and lipoprotein(a), and in raising HDL ("good") cholesterol.[9]

Not only can niacin improve cholesterol levels, it has also been shown to improve overall mortality.

How Does Niacin Work?

As with garlic and many other treatments for high cholesterol, we don't really know how niacin works. Laboratory research has suggested a couple of different theories to explain how niacin lowers cholesterol.

One theory is that niacin affects the release of fats into the bloodstream by altering the function of a crucial enzyme.[10] Another theory is that niacin specifically blocks a process that removes HDL from the blood, thereby raising the HDL level. However, neither of these theories has been fully proven valid.

Dosage

The adult recommended intake of niacin is 16 mg for most men and 14 mg for most women. Cholesterol-lowering doses are much higher, up to 4,000 mg daily.

When using it to reduce cholesterol levels, you should start niacin at a low dose and gradually increase it over several weeks. For example, begin with 50 to 100 mg 3 times daily taken with or just after meals. Increase the dose 100 to 250 mg every 7 to 14 days. According to one study, a minimum dose of 1,000 mg a day is necessary to get the cholesterol-lowering effect with niacin,[11] but many people require somewhat more. A typical dose is 500 to 1,000 mg 3 times daily. Dosages up to 6 to 9 g have been used, but the larger the dose the greater the risk of side effects.

Niacin is more effective than statin drugs in lowering triglycerides and lipoprotein(a), and in raising HDL ("good") cholesterol.

Warning: Don't take niacin in cholesterol-lowering doses without medical supervision. At those high doses, niacin is a drug, not a dietary supplement. Keep in mind that even the starting dose of niacin is about ten times more than you need for good nutrition. While you're on niacin therapy, your doctor will want to periodically check your blood liver enzymes to head off any possible liver toxicity—niacin's most serious potential side effect (see Safety Issues).

The first thing you will notice within 15 minutes to 2 hours of taking niacin is its most common side effect: a skin reaction called *flushing*. Knowing in advance that it's not dangerous does not make it any more comfortable. Prepare for your face and body to turn a shade of red, along with heat sensations, tingling, headache, and itching. You may experience one or more of these symptoms.

In order to reduce flushing, it's best to build up slowly, starting with a moderate dose and increasing it over several weeks, as described previously. Taking aspirin about 30 minutes before niacin can also inhibit the flushing effect. One study showed that taking 325 mg of aspirin before taking niacin reduced flushing, itching, and tingling by as much as 58%.[12] Aspirin inhibits chemicals in the body called *prostaglandins*, which are responsible for the flushing and perhaps some of the other symptoms. Consult your doctor before starting on aspirin or other similar medication in conjunction with niacin.

> To minimize flushing, it's best to build up slowly, starting with a moderate dose and increasing it over several weeks.

Types of Niacin

Another thing to consider when taking niacin is the form you use. Currently, there are three forms of niacin that lower cholesterol. They are ordinary, immediate-release niacin; "flush-free" niacin (developed in Europe and known as *inositol hexaniacinate*); and slow-release niacin.

Most of the scientific research has been on immediate-release niacin. This is the type you are likely to find at your local pharmacy or health-food store. It is definitely effective and very inexpensive.

Inositol hexaniacinate, also called "flush-free" niacin, was developed in Europe as an alternative to standard niacin. It appears to produce less flushing than regular niacin,[13] but flushing still does occur. Inositol hexaniacinate is also said to be safer for the liver, but this hasn't been proven. This "alternative" form of niacin has been suggested as a treatment for other conditions as well. See *The Natural Pharmacist: Your Complete Guide to Vitamins and Supplements* for more information.

Slow-release niacin is available over-the-counter or by prescription. It produces less flushing, but it is possibly more likely to cause liver inflammation than ordinary immediate-release niacin.

Make sure not to buy *niacinamide* by mistake. As a low-dose supplement for general nutrition, niacinamide is identical to niacin and doesn't cause flushing. But high-dose niacinamide does not seem to lower cholesterol.

Be careful to read the labels of the different niacin products to make sure that you get just the form you want.

> **Niacinamide has many nutritional benefits, but it doesn't lower cholesterol. Be careful to read the labels of the different niacin products to make sure that you get the right form.**

Safety Issues

So far, we've heard all the good news about niacin. But it also has a downside. At the beginning of this chapter, we saw that niacin was once a leading conventional treatment for high cholesterol, but it was largely abandoned in favor of the statin drugs. One main reason for this was that niacin produces a number of uncomfortable minor side effects, and some potentially serious risks associated with a particular slow-release form of niacin. The side effects can be troublesome enough to discourage some people from taking niacin. Nonetheless, if you use the proper form of niacin at the right dose, you can often avoid these problems.

John's Story

At age 63, John's cholesterol was moderately high, at 235 mg/dL. Being very conscious of his health, he wanted to get it under control right away before any future problems could develop.

John was already practicing good health habits. He ate a good balance of nutrients and got plenty of fiber. He and his wife were avid walkers who spent at least 30 minutes almost every night walking in their neighborhood. John did some research to see what else might help lower his cholesterol and read some articles about garlic. After discussing it with his doctor, he began taking a standardized garlic extract and including more garlic in his diet.

After about 3 months, John visited his doctor to check on his cholesterol level. To their mutual dismay, it had only

Side Effects

The most common side effect is "flushing," as described previously. This effect occurs in as many as 50% of people who try niacin. Flushing is not dangerous, but it can be uncomfortable and annoying. Fortunately, it seems to decrease over time as the body gets used to its daily dose of niacin. Flushing can be increased by alcohol consumption as well as by the alcohol-deterrent drug disulfiram (Antabuse). (Alcohol can also increase the chance of liver damage with niacin. See following discussion for more on this.)

Aside from flushing, people taking niacin may experience other uncomfortable side effects. About 1 in 4 people taking niacin experience nausea or intestinal prob-

dropped slightly, to 230 mg/dL. John wanted to try a more aggressive approach. His doctor suggested that he begin taking niacin in addition to the garlic, at a dose of 250 mg 3 times a day to start, and gradually work up to twice that dosage. John's doctor also warned him about niacin's side effects and said he should call if he had any problems.

John definitely noticed the flushing at first, but then it subsided. He had no other side effects. After 6 weeks, his doctor rechecked his lipid profile, and this time they were both very pleased. His cholesterol had fallen to 194 mg/dL and his HDL had increased by 20%. His doctor continued to monitor him for his lipids and liver enzymes, and there were no sign of liver problems throughout the course of his treatment.

lems. Dry skin, rash, numbness and tingling of the arms and legs, insomnia, and low blood pressure have all been reported at lower, but still significant, rates of incidence—around 5 to 10% of people taking niacin. The research on niacin tends to show that higher dosages produce more side effects.

Liver Problems

Besides the relatively minor side effects described previously, niacin can cause one serious health problem: liver inflammation or even outright damage. This side effect occurs in about 2 to 6% of individuals taking niacin. Some but not all studies have found that slow-release niacin is more likely to cause this problem than quick-release niacin.[14,15] It appears that the exact form of slow-release niacin plays a role. In addition, a single nightly dose may be safer.

The good news is that liver problems are generally mild and go away when you stop taking niacin. However, there have been four reports of liver failure associated with niacin use; all of these people took slow-release niacin.[16] One person required a liver transplant.

If you use the proper form of niacin at the right dose, you can often avoid side effects and other health risks.

Liver toxicity has appeared after as little as 1 week of therapy and up to as long as 48 months after therapy began.

Flu-like symptoms can be a warning sign of liver problems. These include malaise, fatigue, weakness, sleepiness, appetite loss, nausea, vomiting, stomach pain, and dark urine.[17] However, it is better to catch liver problems early, which can only be accomplished through regular blood tests.

Warning: Because niacin can be hard on the liver, anyone with active liver disease (such as hepatitis or cirrhosis), or a history of liver disease, should avoid niacin completely. The effects could be potentially fatal. People who drink large amounts of alcohol on a regular basis should avoid niacin for the same reason.

Drug Interactions

There are concerns that niacin should not be taken along with statin drugs. The combination might cause increased risk of *rhabdomyolysis*, a condition of severe muscle destruction that can lead to kidney failure. For this reason, it also may not be advisable to combine niacin with red yeast rice, a natural treatment (described in chapter 4) that contains substances in the statin family. However, some evidence suggests that it may be acceptable to combine niacin and statins under close physician supervision.[18,19] As mentioned previously, disulfiram (Antabuse), a drug used to treat alcoholism, may intensify the flushing side effect of niacin, so avoid this combination.

Other Warnings

Niacin is an effective treatment for high cholesterol in people with diabetes. Contrary to previous reports, niacin does not appear to raise blood sugar levels in individuals with diabetes.[20]

Niacin should not be used by individuals with gout; a tendency to form kidney stones, peptic ulcers, or other stomach problems; or a history of liver disease.

Niacin should not be used by individuals with gout or a tendency to form kidney stones.[21]

Many types of digestive complaints have been attributed to niacin use, so people with peptic ulcers or other stomach problems (such as heartburn, nausea, or vomiting) should stay away from niacin.

Warning: As mentioned previously, adding niacin to an already compromised liver could be potentially fatal.

As with many herbs, medications, and nutritional supplements, niacin's safety for pregnant and nursing women is unknown.

Should Children Take Niacin?

One study examined niacin as a cholesterol-lowering treatment for children.[22] This study showed that niacin was effective in reducing total cholesterol and LDL ("bad") cholesterol. However, 76% of the children experienced side effects, and 29% had elevated liver enzymes, indicating that their livers had been irritated or damaged. Based on this study, we don't recommend niacin for children except as a last resort and under the close supervision of a pediatrician.

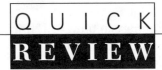

QUICK REVIEW

- High-dose niacin treatment is a well-established, effective method of reducing cholesterol and improving blood lipid profiles. Before the statin drugs were developed, niacin was a leading conventional treatment for high cholesterol. However, due to the potential for liver damage, high-dose niacin should be used only under the supervision of a physician.

- Niacin typically reduces LDL ("bad") cholesterol by approximately 10%, lowers triglycerides by 25%, raises HDL ("good") cholesterol by 20 to 30%, and decreases lipoprotein(a) by about 35%.

- The usual starting dose for niacin is 50 to 100 mg taken 3 times a day with meals. Increase the dose 100 to 250 mg every 7 to 14 days. According to one study, a minimum dose of 1,000 mg a day is necessary for the cholesterol-lowering effect, but for some people, higher doses may be needed. However, the higher the dose, the greater the possible side effects.

- The most common side effect with niacin is "flushing"—a sensation of heat, often combined with redness in the face, headache, or tingling and itching. Flushing is annoying but harmless, and it often decreases after niacin has been taken regularly for awhile.

- A more serious potential health risk with niacin is liver damage. Slow-release niacin has been most prominently associated with liver damage and failure, but other forms of niacin may cause it as well.

- Niacin should not be combined with alcohol or disulfiram (Antabuse). Combination therapy with statin drugs requires close physician supervision.

CHAPTER

FOUR

Other Evidence-Based Natural Treatments for High Cholesterol

his chapter introduces five treatments for high cholesterol that have a significant level of evidence behind them: stanols, soy, policosanol, red yeast rice, and artichoke leaf. Both stanols and soy have been approved by the FDA as "heart healthy," indicating that a diet including either of these substances may reduce the risk of heart disease. Policosanol is not well known but may be as effective as statin drugs. Red yeast rice is a natural source of statin drugs, and also appears to be highly effective. Artichoke leaf is most commonly used for digestive upset, but one moderately large double-blind trial found it helpful for reducing cholesterol.

Stanols

Stanols are substances that occur naturally in various plants. Their cholesterol-lowering effects were first observed in animals in the 1950s. Since then, a substantial amount of research suggests that stanols can help lower cholesterol in individuals with normal or mildly to moderately elevated cholesterol levels. They can also be combined with statin drugs for enhanced effect.

A substantial amount of research suggests that stanols can help lower cholesterol in individuals with normal or mildly to moderately elevated cholesterol levels.

Stanols occur naturally in wood pulp, tall oil, and soybean oil. Stanols are also made commercially from related substances in plants called sterols, such as beta-sitosterol; the resulting substances are sometimes called sitostanols.[1,2] For incorporation into foods, stanols are processed with fatty acids from vegetable oils to form chemicals called stanol esters.[3]

Recently, the FDA has allowed manufacturers of products containing stanols to claim that they are heart healthy. There are several margarines on the market today that are enriched with stanols. Stanols are also added to some salad dressings and other food products, and are available as dietary supplement tablets.

Stanols are thought to work by interfering with the body's ability to absorb cholesterol.[4,5]

What Is the Scientific Evidence for Stanols?

At least 13 double-blind placebo-controlled studies, ranging in length from 30 days to 12 months and involving a total of more than 935 individuals, have found stanols effective for improving cholesterol levels.[6–18] The combined results suggest that stanols can reduce total cholesterol and LDL ("bad") cholesterol by about 10 to 15%. Stanols do not seem to have any consistent effect on HDL ("good") cholesterol or triglycerides.[19]

In one of the best of the double-blind placebo-controlled studies, 153 individuals with mildly elevated cholesterol were given sitostanol esters in margarine (at 1.8 or 2.6 g of sitostanol per day), or margarine without sitostanol ester, for 1 year.[20] The results in the treated group receiving 2.6 g per day showed improvements in total cholesterol by 10.2% and LDL cholesterol by 14.1%—significantly better than the results in the control group. Neither triglycerides nor HDL cholesterol levels were affected.

Stanols are thought to work by interfering with the body's ability to absorb cholesterol.

Two studies have also found that taking stanols along with statin drugs increases the overall cholesterol-lowering effect.[21,22] This makes sense, because stanols reduce absorption of cholesterol from food, while statin drugs stop the body from making its own cholesterol.

In one of these studies, 167 men and women were enrolled who had been taking statin drugs for at least 3 months. None had achieved perfect cholesterol control. For 8 weeks, each participant consumed either 3 servings per day of a stanol ester spread or a placebo spread.

The results were positive. In the treated group, total cholesterol fell by an additional 12% and LDL fell by 17%. Individuals given placebo spread, on the other hand, experienced significantly much smaller improvements. Benefits from the stanol ester spread were seen at 2 weeks, and increased as the study progressed.

Dosage

Typical dosages of stanol esters to lower cholesterol levels range from 3.4 to 5.1 g per day.[23] In terms of margarine spreads, this typically works out to about 3 teaspoons per day. Be patient! It may take up to 3 months to show a substantial decrease in total cholesterol values.[24]

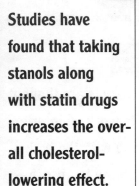

> **Studies have found that taking stanols along with statin drugs increases the overall cholesterol-lowering effect.**

Safety Issues

Stanols are considered safe because they are not absorbed.[25,26] No adverse effects have been reported in any of the studies on lowering cholesterol, with the exception of one study that reported mild gastrointestinal complaints in a few preschool children.[27] In addition, no toxic signs were observed in rats given stanol esters for 13 weeks at levels comparable to or exceeding those recommended for lowering cholesterol.[28]

Although concerns have been expressed that stanols might impair absorption of the fat-soluble vitamins A, D, and E, this does not seem to occur at the dosages of stanols required to lower cholesterol.[29] Stanols might, however, interfere with absorption of alpha- and beta-carotene,[30,31] although some studies have found no such effect.[32,33] Until more is learned, it may be reasonable for individuals using stanol products to make sure to consume plenty of carotenoid-rich vegetables (yellow/orange and dark green vegetables).[34]

Soy

The soybean has been prized for centuries in Asia as a nutritious, high-protein food with myriad uses, and today it's

Marilyn's Story

Marilyn had been taking the medication lovastatin (Mevacor) for 2 years. Although this powerful statin drug had improved her cholesterol level, her LDL cholesterol was still too high.

In 1999, a margarine containing stanols came on the market. Her doctor suggested that she try using some three times a day, instead of butter.

Within a month, her LDL cholesterol had dropped to safe levels. The combination of the two treatments was just what Marilyn needed.

---

popular in the United States, not only in Asian food but also as a cholesterol-free meat and dairy substitute in traditional American foods. Soy burgers, soy yogurt, tofu hot dogs, and tofu cheese can be found in a growing number of grocery stores alongside the traditional white blocks of tofu.

Soy may have many health benefits, including reducing cholesterol levels and preventing some forms of cancer. The FDA has authorized allowing foods containing soy to carry a "heart healthy" label.

We don't really know how soy reduces cholesterol. One theory focuses on constituents of soybeans called isoflavones. These substances act somewhat like estrogen and might be the active ingredients in soy; however, not all evidence agrees.

What Is the Scientific Evidence for Soy?

According to the combined evidence of numerous studies, soy can reduce blood cholesterol levels and improve the ratio of LDL to HDL cholesterol.[35] At an average dosage of 47 g daily, total cholesterol falls by about 9%, LDL cholesterol by 13%, and triglycerides by 10%. Soy may or may not improve HDL cholesterol levels; study results are conflicting.

Soy may have many health benefits, including reducing cholesterol levels and preventing some forms of cancer.

One study found evidence that the isoflavones in soy are the active cholesterol-lowering ingredient.[36] However, other studies suggest that there may be additional constituents in soy that are equally or more important.[37,38]

One indisputable benefit from eating soy is that, unlike animal sources of protein, it contains no saturated fat. However, soy appears to produce benefits above and beyond substituting for less healthful forms of protein.[39]

Dosage

The FDA suggests a daily minimum intake of 25 g of soy protein to reduce cholesterol, although higher intake is probably more effective. This amount is typically found in about 2 1/2 cups of soy milk or 1/2 pound of tofu.

If you like Japanese, Chinese, Thai, or Vietnamese food, it's easy to get a healthy dose of soy. Tofu is one of the world's most versatile foods. It can be stir-fried, steamed, or added to soup. You can also mash a cake of tofu and use it in place of ricotta cheese in your lasagna. If you don't like tofu, there are many other soy products to try: plain soybeans, soy cheese, soy burgers, soy milk, or tempeh. Or you can use a soy supplement instead.

Safety Issues

As a widely eaten food, soy is assumed to be safe. However, there are a few concerns.

Soy may impair thyroid function or reduce absorption of thyroid medication, at least in children.[40,41,42] For this reason, individuals with impaired thyroid function should use soy with caution.

Soy also may reduce the absorption of zinc, iron, and calcium.[43–47] To avoid absorption problems, you should probably take these nutrients at least 2 hours apart from eating soy.

There are some concerns about the isoflavones in soy as well. Studies in animals have found soy isoflavones essentially nontoxic.[48] However, the isoflavones in soy could conceivably have some potentially harmful hormonal effects in certain specific situations. For example, while soy is thought to reduce cancer risk, we don't know if high doses of soy are

> **According to the combined evidence of numerous studies, soy can reduce blood cholesterol levels and improve the ratio of LDL to HDL cholesterol.**

safe for women who have already had breast cancer. Preliminary studies and reports have suggested the possibility that intensive use of soy products by pregnant women could exert a hormonal effect that impacts unborn children.[49,50] Finally, fears have been expressed by some experts that soy might interfere with the action of oral contraceptives. However, one study of 40 women suggests that such concerns are groundless.[51] Another trial found that soy does not interfere with the action of estrogen-replacement therapy in menopausal women.[52]

Seth's Story

Seth didn't believe in taking either drugs or herbs. "I just hate putting pills in my mouth," he would say. Unfortunately, even though he exercised regularly and ate reasonably well, his cholesterol levels were a little on the high side.

A friend suggested Seth add more soy foods to his diet, but he resisted. Seth's reluctance earned him a bit of a lecture. "If you won't take pills and won't eat food that will help lower your cholesterol, then what you're saying is 'I'm not willing to do anything to get better. I want to have a heart attack,'" his friend warned.

Finally, motivated by his friend's concern, Seth decided to take action. He attended a cooking class at the local recreation center, and gradually incorporated 50 g of soy protein daily into his diet. After several months, his cholesterol levels had dropped to within the normal range.

Policosanol

Although it is not well known, the supplement policosanol appears to be a highly effective treatment for elevated cholesterol, perhaps as powerful as statin drugs. This supplement is a mixture of naturally occurring waxy substances manufactured from sugarcane. A substantial amount of research, most of it from Cuba, suggests that policosanol can reduce total and LDL cholesterol levels. Interestingly, nearly all these studies involved individuals for whom dietary change failed to control cholesterol levels. That these individuals responded well to policosanol suggests policosanol, unlike garlic, is more effective than dietary changes.

Policosanol is thought to work by slowing down cholesterol synthesis in the liver and also increasing liver reabsorption of LDL cholesterol.[53,54]

What Is the Scientific Evidence for Policosanol?

Many double-blind studies, involving a total of almost 1,500 individuals and ranging in length from 6 weeks to 12 months, have found policosanol effective for improving cholesterol levels.[55–72] The results suggest that policosanol treatment can reduce LDL cholesterol by 20% or more, and lower total cholesterol by about 15%. Some studies found improvements in HDL cholesterol, but others did not.

Policosanol is thought to work by slowing down cholesterol synthesis in the liver and also increasing liver reabsorption of LDL cholesterol.

In the most recent study, 244 postmenopausal women with high cholesterol received either placebo or policosanol at 5 mg per day for 12 weeks.[73] Then, the dosage was doubled to 10 mg per day (in the treated group) and the study continued for an additional 12 weeks.

The results showed significant improvements in the treated group, with better results when the higher dose was used. At the end of the study, LDL cholesterol improved by 25.2%, total cholesterol by 16.7%, and HDL cholesterol by 27.2%; this was substantially more improvement than what was seen in the placebo group.

Almost identical results were seen in a study of similar design and length following 437 individuals with hyperlipidemia.[74]

In addition, small double-blind trials comparing policosanol against the standard drugs pravastatin, simvastatin and lovastatin have found it equally effective as the medications.[75–79]

Studies have found policosanol safe and effective for reducing cholesterol levels in individuals with type 2 (adult-onset) diabetes.[80,81] However, individuals with any form of diabetes should seek medical advice before taking policosanol.

> **The results of double-blind studies suggest policosanol treatment can reduce LDL cholesterol by 20% or more.**

Dosage

Typical dosages of policosanol to lower elevated cholesterol levels range from 5 to 10 mg twice daily. Results may require 2 months to develop.[82,83]

Safety Issues

Policosanol appears to be safe at the maximum recommended dose. In the double-blind trials described above, only mild, short-term side effects were seen, such as nervousness, headache, diarrhea, and insomnia. In a study that followed 27,879 participants for 2 to 4 years, policosanol produced adverse effects in only 0.31%, primarily weight loss, excessive urination, and insomnia.[84]

No signs of toxicity were observed in animals given very high doses of policosanol (as much as 620 times the maximum recommended dose).[85–88] In addition, the evidence of one human trial suggests that policosanol does not affect the liver.[89] However, safety in young children, pregnant or nursing women, or individuals with severe liver or kidney disease has not been established.

Policosanol has been found not to interact with three types of medications used for high blood pressure: calcium-channel antagonists, diuretics, and beta-blockers.[90] However, policosanol does appear to enhance the blood-thinning effects of aspirin,[91] suggesting that combination therapy could be dangerous. On the same principle, policosanol should not be combined with other blood-thinning drugs, such as aspirin, warfarin (Coumadin), heparin, or pentoxifylline (Trental). There is also at least a remote chance that it might cause excessive bleeding if combined with natural supplements that thin the blood, such as garlic, ginkgo, and high-dose vitamin E. In addition, policosanol might interact unfavorably with the medication levodopa, used for Parkinson's disease.[92] Finally, for theoretical reasons, these sup-

Red yeast rice contains at least 11 naturally occurring substances similar to prescription drugs in the statin family.

plements should not be combined with standard cholesterol-lowering medications except on the advice of a physician.

Red Yeast Rice: Related to the Statin Drugs

Red yeast rice is a traditional Chinese substance that is made by fermenting a type of yeast called *Monascus purpureus* over rice. This product (called Hong Qu) has been used in China since at least 800 A.D. as a food and also as a medicinal substance. Recently, it has been discovered that this ancient Chinese preparation contains at least 11 naturally occurring substances similar to prescription drugs in the statin family. However, a normal dose of red yeast rice contains rather low concentrations of these substances. For this reason, it is thought that various statin components and perhaps other constituents of red yeast rice work in concert to lower cholesterol levels.

What Is the Scientific Evidence for Red Yeast Rice?

A U.S. study on red yeast rice was conducted at the UCLA School of Medicine.[93] This was a 12-week double-blind placebo-controlled trial involving 83 healthy participants (46 men and 37 women, aged 34 to 78 years) with high cholesterol levels. One group was given the recommended dose of red yeast rice, while the other group received placebo. Both groups were instructed to consume a lowfat diet similar to the American Heart Association Step 1 diet.

The results showed that red yeast rice was significantly more effective than placebo. In the treated group, average total cholesterol fell by about 18% by 8 weeks. During the same time period, LDL cholesterol decreased by 22% and triglycerides by 11%. There was little to no improvement in the placebo group. HDL cholesterol did not change in either group during the study.

Similar or even better results have been seen in other U.S. and Chinese studies using various forms of red yeast rice.[94,95]

Dosage

Because red yeast rice products can vary widely in their strength, please refer to the labeling for appropriate dosage.

Safety Issues

While there have been no serious adverse reactions reported in the studies of red yeast rice, some minor side effects have been reported. In a large open trial in which 324 people received red yeast rice, heartburn (1.8%), bloating (0.9%), and dizziness (0.3%) were all mentioned.[96] Formal toxicity studies in rats and mice, giving doses up to 125 times the normal human dose for 3 months, showed no toxic effects, according to information published by one of the manufacturers of red yeast rice.[97]

Because red yeast rice contains ingredients similar to the statin drugs, there is a theoretical risk of the same side effects and risks that are seen with those drugs. These include elevated liver enzymes, damage to skeletal muscle, and increased risk of cancer. Also, red yeast rice should not be combined with erythromycin, statin drugs, the class of drugs called "fibrates," or, perhaps, high-dose niacin.

Additionally, like statin drugs, red yeast rice may deplete the body of a substance called coenzyme Q_{10} (CoQ_{10}).[98–101] Taking extra CoQ_{10} might be helpful. (See chapter 7 for more information on CoQ_{10}.)

Grapefruit juice can cause a significant and possibly dangerous increase in blood levels of statin drugs. For this reason, grapefruit juice should be avoided when taking red yeast rice.

This product should not be used by pregnant or nursing women or people with severe liver or kidney disease except on a physician's advice.

Artichoke Leaf

The artichoke is one of the oldest cultivated plants. It was first grown in Ethiopia and then made its way to southern Europe via Egypt. Its image is found on ancient Egyptian tablets and sacrificial altars. The ancient Greeks and Romans considered it a valuable digestive aid and reserved what was then a rare plant for consumption in elite circles. In sixteenth-century Europe, the artichoke was also considered a "noble" vegetable meant for consumption by the royal and the rich.

In traditional European medicine, the leaves of the artichoke (not the flower buds, which are the parts commonly cooked and eaten as a vegetable) were used as a diuretic to stimulate the kidneys and as a "choleretic" to stimulate the flow of bile from the liver and gallbladder. (Bile is a yellowish-brown fluid manufactured in the liver and stored in the gallbladder; it consists of numerous substances, including several that play a significant role in digestion.)

Artichoke leaf is used in Germany today to improve digestion. However, there is actually better evidence that artichoke can lower cholesterol levels. Artichoke leaf may work by interfering with cholesterol synthesis.[102] A compound in artichoke called luteolin may play a role in reducing cholesterol.[103]

What Is the Scientific Evidence for Artichoke Leaf?

According to a double-blind placebo-controlled study of 143 individuals with elevated cholesterol, artichoke leaf extract significantly improved cholesterol readings.[104] Total cholesterol fell by 18.5% as compared to 8.6% in the placebo group; LDL cholesterol fell by 23% versus 6%; and the LDL to HDL ratio decreased by 20% versus 7%.

Artichoke leaf is used in Germany today to improve digestion, but there is better evidence that it can lower cholesterol levels.

Dosage

Germany's Commission E recommends 6 g of the dried artichoke leaf (or an amount of extract equivalent to it) per day, usually divided into 3 doses.

Safety Issues

Artichoke leaf has not been associated with significant side effects in studies so far, but full safety testing has not been completed. For this reason, it should not be used by pregnant or nursing women. Safety in young children or in people with severe liver or kidney disease has also not been established.

In addition, because artichoke leaf is believed to stimulate gallbladder contraction, individuals with gallstones or other forms of gallbladder disease could be put at risk by using this herb. Such individuals should use artichoke leaf only under the supervision of a physician. It is possible that increased gallbladder contraction could lead to obstruction of ducts or even rupture of the gallbladder.

Individuals with known allergies to artichokes or related plants in the Asteraceae family, such as arnica or chrysanthemums, should avoid using artichoke.

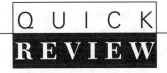

QUICK
REVIEW

- The combined results of at least 13 double-blind placebo-controlled studies suggest that stanols can reduce total cholesterol and LDL cholesterol by about 10 to 15%.

- Recently, the FDA has allowed manufacturers of products containing stanols to claim that they are heart healthy. There are several margarines on the market today that are enriched with stanols. Stanols are also added to some salad dressings and other food products, and are available as dietary supplement tablets.

- Soy may have many health benefits, including reducing cholesterol levels and preventing some forms of cancer. However, there are some safety concerns.

- The results of many studies suggest that treatment with policosanol, a supplement manufactured from sugarcane, can reduce cholesterol about as much as drugs in the statin family. Policosanol should not be combined with drugs that thin the blood, such as aspirin, warfarin (Coumadin), heparin, and pentoxifylline (Trental). Combination therapy with natural blood thinners, such as garlic, ginkgo, and vitamin E, might also be risky. Finally, policosanol might interfere with the Parkinson's disease medication levodopa.

- Red yeast rice is a promising treatment for high cholesterol. You should refer to the package labeling for the proper dosage. Because it contains ingredients similar to those of statin drugs, the same safety warnings for those medications also apply to red yeast rice.

- Artichoke leaf may lower cholesterol by interfering with cholesterol synthesis. A compound in artichoke called luteolin may also play a role. Since artichoke leaf is believed to stimulate gallbladder contraction, people with gallstones or other forms of gallbladder disease should probably not take artichoke.

Other Supplements for High Cholesterol

I n addition to the treatments discussed thus far, other dietary supplements are available that might help reduce cholesterol levels. While none of these have very strong scientific documentation as yet, many do have preliminary evidence in their favor and offer considerable promise.

Gugulipid: A Traditional Indian Herb

Gugulipid is the standardized extract derived from the bark of the Mukul myrrh tree *(Commiphora mukul),* a small, thorny tree native to India and Arabia. This substance has been used for thousands of years as part of a traditional Indian medical system called *Ayurveda.* It appears to reduce total cholesterol by about 12%, lower LDL ("bad") cholesterol by 12 to 17%, and increase HDL ("good") cholesterol by a similar amount.

The main constituents of gugulipid are substances called *guggulsterones*. Both E-guggulsterone and Z-guggulsterone are believed (but not proven) to be the active ingredients. We don't know how gugulipid works. One study in rats suggests that guggulsterones cause the liver to remove LDL from the blood.[1]

What Is the Scientific Evidence for Gugulipid?

A double-blind placebo-controlled study investigated the effect of dietary modification and gugulipid on cholesterol levels in 61 people.[2] After 12 weeks of following a healthy diet, half the participants received placebo and the other half received guggul at a dose providing 100 mg of guggulsterones daily. The results after 24 weeks of treatment showed that the treated group experienced an 11.7% decrease in total cholesterol, along with a 12.7% decrease in LDL ("bad") cholesterol, a 12% decrease in triglycerides, and an 11.1% decrease in the total cholesterol/HDL ("good") cholesterol ratio. These improvements were significantly greater than what was seen in the placebo group.

Gugulipid is a substance that has been used for thousands of years as part of a traditional Indian medical system called *Ayurveda*.

Similar results were seen in a placebo-controlled trial of 40 individuals (the study report didn't state whether or not it was double-blind).[3]

Finally, a double-blind crossover study compared the effects of gugulipid with the fibric acid drug clofibrate (described in more detail in chapter 7).[4] Two hundred and thirty-three people were enrolled in the study. The average total cholesterol was 258 mg/dL in the gugulipid group and 281 mg/dL in the clofibrate group. Both groups took 500 mg 3 times a day of either gugulipid or clofibrate for a period of 12 weeks. Afterward, there was a brief washout period (during which neither group received any treatment), then the two groups' treatments were switched for an additional 8 weeks.

In this study, gugulipid was more effective than clofibrate at improving cholesterol levels. Although clofibrate decreased total cholesterol slightly more than gugulipid (15% versus 13%), gugulipid had more of an effect on LDL cholesterol, which is probably more important than total cholesterol. LDL dropped 17% in participants taking gugulipid versus a 13% decrease in the clofibrate group. HDL also increased significantly in the gugulipid group (16%), while the clofibrate group did not see a change that was statistically significant.

Dosage

Most of the clinical studies have used a product standardized to contain 5 to 10% guggulsterones, taken at a dose of 500 mg 3 times a day. The course of treatment should be 3 to 6 months.

Safety Issues

Based on animal toxicity studies, gugulipid appears to be quite safe. In 6-month toxicity studies in rats, monkeys, and beagles, gugulipid showed no adverse effects.[5,6] In a toxicity study using mice, the LD_{30} (the dose needed to kill 30% of the mice) was 1,600 mg per kilogram body weight, or roughly 50 times the recommended dose.[7]

In clinical trials of standardized guggul extract, no significant side effects other than occasional mild gastrointestinal distress have been seen.[8,9,10] Laboratory tests conducted in the course of these trials did not reveal any alterations in liver or kidney function, blood cell numbers

James's Story

James, 73, had recently been diagnosed with high cholesterol and triglycerides, despite maintaining an active lifestyle and eating a fairly healthy diet. He was surprised that his total cholesterol was 266 mg/dL even though he had always worked hard to take care of himself. He requested an aggressive treatment, so his doctor suggested he take a standardized garlic supplement, 1,500 mg of niacin, and 1,500 mg of standardized gugulipid daily. James was to stay on this regimen for at least 3 months.

At his follow-up visit, his cholesterol level had improved dramatically: It had dropped to 190 mg/dL. Both James and

and appearance, heart function, or blood chemistry. However, there haven't been any long-term safety studies in humans.

There are no known interactions between gugulipid and drugs, although this doesn't mean that some won't be reported eventually. Safety in young children, pregnant or nursing women, or those with severe liver or kidney disease has not been established.

Pantethine: Particularly Effective for Elevated Triglycerides

Pantethine is closely related to pantothenic acid, or vitamin B_5. The name is derived from the Greek word *pantos*, which means "everywhere." Indeed, vitamin B_5 can be found in virtually every type of food. It is a major component of a molecule called *coenzyme A* (CoA), which is important because it is involved in many biochemical

his doctor were very pleased with the results. James did have some temporary difficulties with the niacin, but his body soon adapted, and he was able to stay on his cholesterol-lowering regimen. (For a more detailed discussion of niacin's side effects, see chapter 3.)

Since James used three treatments at once, it is not possible to say which of them helped him most, or whether it was the combination that worked. We really need studies that evaluate the safety and effectiveness of these natural treatments when used together.

pathways and is responsible for the transport of fats in and out of cells. For reasons that are not clear, pantethine supplements (but not pantothenic acid supplements) appear to reduce levels of both triglycerides and cholesterol.

What Is the Scientific Evidence for Pantethine?

According to a few small studies, pantethine can strikingly lower triglyceride levels and improve total and LDL cholesterol.

One double-blind placebo-controlled study examined 29 individuals with elevated cholesterol and triglycerides.[11] For 8 weeks, participants were given either 300 mg of pantethine 3 times daily or placebo; then treatments were switched for an additional 8 weeks. In this study, subjects taking pantethine experienced a 30% reduction in blood triglycerides, a 13.5% reduction in LDL cholesterol, and a 10% rise in HDL cholesterol, a significant improvement compared to placebo.

Similar benefits were seen in another small controlled trial.[12]

Several open studies have specifically studied the use of pantethine to improve cholesterol and triglyceride levels in people with diabetes and found it effective.[13–16]

According to a few small studies, pantethine can strikingly lower triglyceride levels and improve total and LDL cholesterol.

These findings are supported by experiments in rabbits, which show that pantethine may prevent the buildup of plaque in major arteries.[17]

However, as often happens when studies are very small, two other controlled trials found no benefit.[18,19] Larger and longer double-blind trials are needed to confirm whether pantethine is truly effective.

Dosage

The usual dose of pantethine is 300 mg 3 times daily. Unfortunately, pantethine is expensive. Because of its high price, we recommend pantethine as an alternative only after other less-costly methods have failed to work for you.

Safety Issues

Pantethine appears to be a safe supplement. One long-term study gave 24 individuals 900 mg of pantethine daily for 1 year without any problems.[20] Formal animal toxicity studies have not been done, but there have been no reports of adverse effects in any of the human studies on pantethine.

There are no known drug interactions with pantethine. Safety in pregnant or nursing women or people with severe liver or kidney disease has not been established.

Tocotrienols: Promising, but More Research Is Needed

Tocotrienols are naturally occurring substances that are forms of vitamin E and that may offer some benefit in lowering your cholesterol. They are found in high amounts in palm oil and rice bran oil.

What Is the Scientific Evidence for Tocotrienols?

The few controlled trials on tocotrienols that have been performed in humans have produced varied findings. One researcher evaluated a special mixture of tocotrienols plus vitamin E (alpha-tocopherol) in a double-blind placebo-controlled study of 41 people with high cholesterol levels.[21] Total cholesterol fell by 16% and LDL cholesterol fell by 23% in the treatment group, compared to 7% and 11%, respectively, in the placebo group.

Like statin drugs, tocotrienols seem to inhibit the enzyme HMG-CoA reductase, at least in test tube studies.[22] However, we don't know if this is what tocotrienols actually do when people take them by mouth. More research needs to be done before we can pinpoint with confidence the mechanism for tocotrienols' effect on cholesterol.

Furthermore, another controlled trial found that the same proprietary tocotrienol mixture used in the study just mentioned may help protect against atherosclerosis, but surprisingly, showed no benefit in lowering cholesterol.[23] Fifty individuals with atherosclerosis involving the brain were followed over 18 months. Of the 25 treated participants, plaque deposits appeared to improve in 7 and to progress in 2. None of the 25 participants in the control group showed improvement and 10 showed progression. But there was no change in cholesterol levels in either group. This directly contradicts the first study and leaves us somewhat in the dark as to whether tocotrienols actually work. Larger studies are needed to help sort out this tangle.

Dosage

We don't know enough about tocotrienols to determine the best therapeutic dose. A dose frequently recommended is one to two 25-mg capsules daily. However, in one of the studies just described, a 220-mg tocotrienol mixture was used.

Safety Issues

There have not been any reported side effects or signs of toxicity at the doses used in the studies, but formal safety studies on tocotrienols have not been done. Maximum safe doses have not been determined for pregnant or nursing women or people with severe kidney or liver disease.

Chitosan: A Form of Dietary Fiber

Chitosan is a form of dietary fiber. Like other forms of fiber, such as oat bran,[24] chitosan appears to reduce cholesterol levels.

Fiber is not well digested by the human body. As it passes through the digestive tract, fiber seems to have an ability to bond with ingested fat and carry it out in the stool. This has the effect of reducing cholesterol levels in the blood. (For more information on fiber, see chapter 6.)

Chitosan is extracted from the shells of shrimp, crab, or lobster. It is also found in yeast and some fungi. Another inexpensive source is "squid pens," a by-product of squid processing; these are small, plastic-like, inedible pieces of squid that are removed prior to eating.

What Is the Scientific Evidence for Chitosan?

In one preliminary placebo-controlled crossover study (apparently blinded, but this was not stated), researchers gave biscuits containing chitosan to 8 healthy adult men. The chitosan dose was 3 to 6 g daily during 2 ingestion periods equaling 14 days total over a 4-week time span.[25] Results showed a statistically significant reduction in total cholesterol and an increase in HDL cholesterol as compared to placebo. Cholesterol reduction was also seen in a controlled but unblinded study of 80 individuals with kidney failure.[26]

This research in humans supports evidence previously found in several animal studies.[27–32]

Dosage

The standard dosage of chitosan is 3 to 6 g per day, to be taken with food.

Chitosan can deplete the body of certain minerals (see Safety Issues). For this reason, when using chitosan, it may be helpful to take supplemental calcium, vitamin D, selenium, magnesium, and other minerals.

Also, according to a preliminary study in rats, taking vitamin C along with chitosan might provide additional benefit in lowering cholesterol.[33]

Safety Issues

There is significant evidence that long-term, high-dose chitosan supplementation can result in malabsorption of some crucial vitamins and minerals

Like other forms of fiber, such as oat bran, chitosan appears to reduce cholesterol levels.

including calcium, magnesium, selenium, and vitamins A, D, E, and K.[34,35] In turn, this appears to lead to a risk of osteoporosis in adults and growth retardation in children. For this reason, adults taking chitosan should also take supplemental vitamins and minerals, making especially sure to get enough vitamin D, calcium, and magnesium.

Another possible risk of long-term ingestion of high doses of chitosan is that it could change the intestinal flora and allow the growth of unhealthful bacteria.[36]

Pregnant or nursing women and young children should probably avoid chitosan altogether.

Fish Oil: Reduces Triglycerides

While it is very important to cut down on saturated fat in your diet, certain fats may actually be healthy for you.

Fish contain omega-3 fatty acids, a form of polyunsaturated fat that may be protective against heart disease. Omega-3 fatty acids are "essential fatty acids" that are not made by the body and must be supplied by the diet or by

Fish contain omega-3 fatty acids, a form of polyunsaturated fat that may be protective against heart disease.

supplements. Interest in them began when it was found that natives of northern Canada who lived extensively on fish had few heart attacks despite a very high fat intake.

It appears that the omega-3 fatty acids produce little effect on total cholesterol levels, but significantly decrease triglycerides.[37] They may slightly raise LDL cholesterol, but this effect is usually temporary.

Fish oil may also help prevent blood clots, lower blood pressure, and decrease homocysteine levels (you may recall from chapter 1 that homocysteine is another suspected risk factor for atherosclerosis).[38]

Dosage

Typical dosages of fish oil are 3 to 9 g daily. The most important omega-3 fatty acids found in fish oil are called

EPA (eicosapentaenoic acid) and DHA (docosahexaenoic acid). In order to match the dosage used in several major studies, you should probably take enough fish oil to supply about 1.8 g (1,800 mg) of EPA and 0.9 g (900 mg) of DHA daily. Some manufacturers add vitamin E to fish oil capsules to keep the oil from becoming rancid. Another method is to remove all the oxygen from the capsule.

Flaxseed oil also contains omega-3 fatty acids, although of a different kind. It has been suggested as a less smelly substitute for fish oil. However, there is no evidence that it is effective when used for the same therapeutic purposes as fish oil.[39]

Safety Issues

Fish oil appears to be safe. The most common problem is fishy burps.

Because fish oil has a mild blood-thinning effect, it should not be combined with powerful blood-thinning medications, such as warfarin (Coumadin) or heparin, except on a physician's advice. However, contrary to some reports, fish oil does not seem to cause bleeding problems when it is taken by itself.[40,41]

Also, fish oil does not appear to raise blood sugar levels in people with diabetes.[42] Nonetheless, if you have diabetes, you should not take any supplement except on the advice of a physician.

If you decide to use cod liver oil as your fish oil supplement, make sure you do not exceed the safe maximum intake of vitamin A and vitamin D. These vitamins are fat soluble, which means that excess amounts tend to build up in your body, possibly reaching toxic levels. Pregnant women should not take more than 2,667 IU of vitamin A daily because of the risk of birth defects; 5,000 IU per day is a reasonable upper limit for other individuals. Look at the bottle label to determine how much vitamin A you are receiving. (It is less likely that you will get enough vitamin D to produce toxic effects.)

Aortic Glycosaminoglycans (GAGs): May Fight Atherosclerosis

Aortic glycosaminoglycans (GAGs) are substances found in high concentrations in the walls of the arteries. Taking GAG supplements may slow the progression of athero-sclerosis and possibly reduce cholesterol levels, although we are not sure how.

Taking GAG sup-plements may slow the progres-sion of atheroscle-rosis and possibly reduce cholesterol levels.

In a recent study, a group of men with early hardening of the coronary arteries was given 200 mg per day of GAGs, while an-other group was not treated.[43] After 18 months, the layering of the vessel lining was 7.5 times greater in the untreated group than in the GAG group, a signif-icant difference. Additional pre-liminary evidence that aortic GAGs might help atherosclerosis comes from other studies in ani-mals and people.[44,45] However, in the absence of properly de-signed double-blind trials, the results can't be taken as truly reliable.

We don't know how aortic GAGs might work. There is some evidence that they can reduce cholesterol levels and thin the blood.[46,47] However, more research is necessary to know for sure.

L-Carnitine: An Expensive Supplement

Another supplement that might show some benefit is L-carnitine. L-carnitine is an amino acid that the body uses to turn fat into energy. It is not normally considered an essential nutrient, since the body can manufacture all it needs. However, supplemental L-carnitine may improve the ability of certain tissues to produce energy. This has led to the use of L-carnitine in various muscle diseases as well as heart conditions.

Weak evidence suggests that L-carnitine may be able to improve cholesterol and triglyceride levels.[48]

Since L-carnitine is very expensive, and there is little evidence as yet that it works, we recommend using other more proven and cost-effective therapies to reduce your cholesterol.

Lecithin: Popular, but No Evidence That It Works

Although there is a widespread belief that lecithin can lower cholesterol, a recent, small, double-blind study of 23 men with high cholesterol levels found that lecithin treatment had no significant effects on total blood cholesterol, triglycerides, HDL cholesterol, LDL cholesterol, or lipoprotein(a).[49] There is little good positive evidence to set against this negative study.

Offsetting Cholesterol-Related Side Effects of Drugs

Medications in the beta-blocker family sometimes reduce levels of HDL cholesterol. One study found that taking supplemental chromium countered this unhealthy side effect.[50] A safe nutritional dose of chromium for adults is 200 mcg daily.

Another positive interaction with a medication involves a combination of vitamins C and E and the drug tamoxifen. Tamoxifen has a tendency to raise triglyceride levels. In one study, simultaneous use of vitamin C (500 mg daily) and vitamin E (400 mg daily) counteracted this side effect.[51]

Miscellaneous Herbs and Supplements

Preliminary evidence suggests possible cholesterol- or triglyceride-lowering benefits with supplemental calcium, probiotics (friendly bacteria), spirulina (a form of algae sold as a dietary supplement), creatine, and alfalfa.[52–76]

Other herbs and supplements commonly recommended for high cholesterol include ashwagandha, bilberry leaf, chondroitin, copper, fenugreek, gamma oryzanol, grass pollen, He shou wu, and maitake, but there is as yet little to no real evidence that they work.

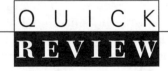

QUICK REVIEW

- Most of the clinical studies of the effectiveness of gugulipid have used a product standardized to contain 5 to 10% guggulsterones, taken at a dose of 500 mg 3 times a day. The course of treatment should be 3 to 6 months.

- According to a few small studies, pantethine can strikingly lower triglyceride levels and improve total and LDL cholesterol. Pantethine is related to pantothenic acid (vitamin B₅), but pantothenic acid does not appear to be effective in improving cholesterol levels. The usual dose of pantethine is 300 mg 3 times daily. Unfortunately, pantethine is expensive.

- Somewhat contradictory evidence also suggests that tocotrienols may be helpful. A dose frequently recommended is one to two 25-mg capsules daily. However, in one study, 220 mg daily of a special tocotrienol mixture was used.

- A dietary form of fiber called chitosan appears to reduce cholesterol levels. The standard dosage of chitosan is 3 to 6 g per day, to be taken with food. However, chitosan can cause malabsorption of calcium, vitamin D, selenium, magnesium, and other minerals. Taking supplements of these minerals may be helpful.

- Other products such as fish oil, aortic glycosaminoglycans, and L-carnitine may be helpful, but more research needs to be done.

- There is no real evidence that lecithin reduces cholesterol levels.

- The mineral chromium and a mixture of vitamins C and E may help offset the cholesterol-related side effects of certain medications.

Lifestyle Changes

There is no doubt that diet, exercise, and healthful lifestyle choices are the cornerstones of good health. This chapter will give you information about specific changes in your diet, exercise habits, and lifestyle that can lower your cholesterol and protect you against cardiovascular disease.

The National Cholesterol Education Program (a government-funded group of scientists) recommends that you try changing your diet, exercise, and lifestyle habits before you consider drug therapy. If you have mild to moderately high cholesterol, you might not need any further treatment to bring your cholesterol to a desirable level. Even if you do end up needing to use a drug or natural supplement to reduce your cholesterol level, you'll get better, longer-lasting results if you combine the treatment with a healthy diet and exercise routine, and, above all, if you give up smoking and excessive drinking. In fact, the benefits of a healthy diet and lifestyle go far beyond merely reducing your cholesterol level. They can improve your health in a number of ways, protecting you not only from heart disease, but from a number of other serious health risks as well.

Quit Smoking

The best advice about smoking is the bluntest: Stop as soon as you can. Good things start to happen in your body soon after you quit. Cigarette smoking is such a widespread and significant risk factor for heart disease that the U.S. Surgeon General has called it "the most important of the known modifiable risk factors for coronary heart disease in the United States."

> **According to the U.S. Surgeon General, cigarette smoking is "the most important of the known modifiable risk factors for coronary heart disease in the United States."**

According to the American Heart Association, a smoker has more than twice a nonsmoker's risk for having a heart attack. Cigarette smoking is the risk factor most associated with sudden cardiac death. Smokers who suffer a heart attack are more likely to die and die suddenly (within 1 hour) than nonsmokers. Evidence also suggests that passive smoking (chronic exposure to secondhand tobacco smoke) may increase the risk of heart disease.

Although we can't tell you that it's easy to quit smoking, we *can* tell you that it's worth the trouble. If you want to quit smoking, consult your doctor for advice and help.

Better Nutrition

With busy work schedules, taking care of the kids, and trying to spend time with friends and family, many people feel they don't have time to cook. Eating on the run, skipping meals, and fast food seem to be the norm in our society. As a result, the quality of our meals has declined.

This isn't to say that you can't lead an active life and still eat a good diet. In fact, it's easier than you might think. Above all, you can improve your diet greatly just by becoming more aware of the food you eat—what's in it and what it does in your body. Even if you never eat at home, you can eat a more healthful diet just by knowing more about the health effects of ordinary foods.

When the subject of making dietary changes comes up, people often ask, "Does this mean I can't eat anything good?" or "Can I still eat my favorite dish?" Relax—making dietary changes is *not* the same as going on a diet. You don't have to give up all the foods you like; what you need to do is to shift your diet as a whole in a generally healthier direction.

For example, someone who eats a lot of steak could try switching some of the time to grilled salmon. The fat you get from beef is saturated fat that will tend to raise your cholesterol, but the fat in salmon (omega-3 fatty acids and other polyunsaturated fats) may actually lower your cholesterol.

A healthy diet doesn't actually mean giving up everything you enjoy.

Sometimes, patients seem to suspect that the entire medical establishment is conspiring to take the fun out of eating. But a healthy diet doesn't actually mean giving up everything you enjoy. As we will see in this chapter, there are specific scientific reasons for the recommendations to consume less saturated fat and meat and more whole grains, legumes, fresh fruits, and vegetables. With practice, you can achieve a healthier diet without sacrificing pleasure.

Reducing Saturated Fats and Increasing Unsaturated Fats

We get two kinds of fat from our food. *Saturated fats* are found in almost anything that contains fat, but are highest in animal products including red meat, whole milk, butter, and lard, and in some vegetable sources, such as palm or coconut oils and vegetable shortening. Because of their chemical structure, saturated fats tend to be opaque or solid at room temperature.

Unsaturated fats are either *monounsaturated*, which means they have only one double bond between carbon molecules, or *polyunsaturated*, which means they have more than one double bond between carbon molecules. Monounsaturated fats are found in large quantities in olive oil, canola oil, and other nut oils. Polyunsaturated fats are found in corn oil, safflower oil, soybean oil, and cold-water fish such as salmon. Both types of unsaturated fats tend to be liquid at room temperature.

For healthier cooking, use monounsaturated fats such as olive oil and canola oil.

Saturated fats seem to be a major culprit in raising cholesterol levels. The unsaturated fats, by contrast, actually seem to lower cholesterol levels.[1,2] Monounsaturated fats may be best for cooking, because they don't break down easily with heat. For healthier cooking, use monounsaturated fats such as olive oil and canola oil. Polyunsaturated fats can be more easily transformed into unhealthy *lipid peroxides* at high temperatures.

A 1997 review of studies tried to determine how dietary fatty acids and cholesterol affected cholesterol in the blood.[3] The authors found that replacing saturated fat with either polyunsaturated fat or monounsaturated fat led to a decline in cholesterol. Reducing dietary cholesterol also resulted in a drop in blood cholesterol. The combined effect from the dietary changes used in these trials was about a 10 to 15% decrease in total cholesterol.

Simply reducing the total amount of fat in your diet can help too. In a 1998 review, 19 controlled studies were evaluated, and the analysis of these trials found that restricting the amount of fat in your diet (to less than 30% of total calories) lowered cholesterol by an average of 6%.[4] However, it's interesting to note that changing the *type* of fat in the diet is more effective than reducing the *total amount* of fat.

Go Nuts on Nuts

A surprisingly large body of evidence suggests that increased consumption of nuts such as almonds, walnuts, pecans, and macadamia nuts may help lower cholesterol and prevent heart disease.[5–12] Like olive oil, nuts contain monounsaturated fats, and this is presumably why they work.

Cut Back on Trans Fatty Acids

Although margarine was introduced on the market as being

Evidence suggests that increased consumption of nuts such as almonds, walnuts, pecans, and macadamia nuts may help lower cholesterol and prevent heart disease.

healthier than butter, this may not be true. Margarine is high in unusual fats called trans fatty acids. These substances seem to *raise* total cholesterol; even worse, they seem to raise LDL ("bad") cholesterol and reduce HDL ("good") cholesterol.[13,14] Any food that contains "hydrogenated" or "partially hydrogenated" oils also contains these unhealthy fats. However, this is a rapidly evolving subject of research, and the last word has not been said on the subject. Interestingly, taking magnesium may help reduce the risks created by margarine.[15] As we discussed in chapter 4, some manufacturers add stanol esters to margarine to help lower your cholesterol.

It appears that adding soluble fiber to your diet can lower cholesterol by about 5 to 15%, depending on the type and amount of fiber used.

Increase Your Intake of Fiber

It has been well documented that a lowfat, high-fiber diet can reduce the risk of certain cancers, particularly colon cancer. Fiber may also lower your cholesterol level.

Dietary fiber is primarily derived from the cell walls of plants. It is especially high in whole, unprocessed grains, fruits and vegetables, and in legumes such as dried beans and lentils. Fiber is important in many functions of the intestinal tract, including digestion and the excretion of wastes. Fiber also removes bile acids from the gut and thus has a mild cholesterol-lowering effect. As we will see in chapter 7, one class of cholesterol-lowering medication—the resin drugs—works on the same principle.

There are two kinds of fiber: *soluble fiber*, which swells up and holds water; and *insoluble fiber*, which does not. Particularly high levels of useful soluble fiber are found in *psyllium* (a plant grown primarily in Asia and India), apples, and oat bran. Insoluble fiber consists mainly of *cellulose*, which is the main constituent of the cell walls in most plants. Most plant-based foods contain insoluble fiber, but wheat bran and flaxseeds are particularly good sources of it. Insoluble fiber seems to provide the best protection against colon cancer, but when it comes to lowering cholesterol, soluble fiber seems to be more effective. One double-blind placebo-controlled study found that psyllium husks reduced LDL cholesterol by 5% over 24 weeks.[16] Although the decrease in LDL was modest, every little bit counts, especially when the treatment is safe.

Other forms of fiber may be more effective. A double-blind placebo-controlled study found that oat bran reduced total cholesterol by 13% more and LDL cholesterol by 17% more than placebo. In the same study, rice bran—a soluble fiber—did almost as well.[17] Other studies have found similar results.[18,19]

Based on these studies, it appears that adding soluble fiber to your diet can lower cholesterol by about 5 to 15%, depending on the type and amount of fiber used. Soluble fiber is found in almost all fruits, vegetables, and legumes. If you take a fiber supplement, the recommended dose is about 10 g daily, with plenty of water.

Exercise, Exercise, Exercise

It has been clearly established over the years that regular exercise can help improve your lipid profile. Based on some studies, it appears that aerobic exercise can lower cholesterol by about 10 to 15%, as well as improve levels of LDL, HDL, and triglycerides.[20,21] Exercise also has many other health benefits: It can help you lose weight; lower your blood pressure; decrease stress; and increase your strength, flexibility, and energy. There is also evidence that regular exercise can help you live longer.[22,23]

The best types of exercise for reducing cholesterol are aerobic exercises such as walking, jogging, bicycling, swimming, or any other activity that gets your heart rate up for a sustained period of time. Aerobic exercise is different from muscle-building activity such as weight lifting. While building muscle also seems to offer health benefits, it is primarily aerobic exercise that reduces cholesterol levels.

The best thing about aerobic exercise is that it is easy to do and doesn't cost a lot of money. You don't have to buy an expensive treadmill or exercise bike. Simply taking brisk walks can be quite beneficial. The key to any successful exercise program is *consistency*. If you only exercise once in a blue moon, you're not likely to see results. But even a modest amount of exercise several times a week can give you results over time.

Expect that it will take some time to build up your endurance, especially if you haven't exercised in awhile.

To get the maximum benefit from aerobic exercise, you need to continue the activity for a sustained time period with moderate intensity. In other words, you should feel like you're working pretty hard, without feeling strained or exhausted. For example, if you choose to go walking, a slow stroll is not as beneficial as walking at a quick pace. However, it is very important that you don't overwork yourself, especially if you're just starting an exercise program. Start slowly and build up your stamina over time.

While no one seems to agree on an exact program for everyone, it appears that moderate aerobic exercise three to five times per week for 15 to 30 minutes can help lower your cholesterol. The trick is finding a type of exercise that is fun for you. Torturing yourself will probably be counterproductive, because you won't keep it up. Choose an activity that you enjoy and that you can manage to do regularly. Also, try to be patient. Many people get frustrated when first starting a program, because the results aren't immediately obvious. Expect that it will take some time to build up your endurance, especially if you haven't exercised in awhile. The same may be true for your cholesterol. Remember, the effects of exercise are cumulative, which means that if you can stay motivated to do it consistently, you are more likely to have your cholesterol drop and stay down.

Remember, the effects of exercise are cumulative. If you can stay motivated to do it consistently, you are more likely to improve your cholesterol level.

Before starting any exercise program, consult your doctor to see whether you have any medical conditions that might limit your choice of exercise. Your physician can also suggest specific activities that might be better for you.

Warning: If at any point during exercise, you begin to experience chest pain, dizziness, or breathlessness, discontinue the activity and consult your physician immediately.

Alcohol: Only in Moderation

Studies suggest that moderate drinking of beer, wine, or spirits can actually reduce the risk of heart disease.[24,25]

In one study, the equivalent of two drinks a day of any kind of alcohol lowered the incidence of heart disease compared to not drinking.[26] But consuming more than two drinks a day resulted in a higher risk of heart attack and stroke. In this study, red wine showed stronger effects

Erik's Story

Erik, 39, works for a large computer company and puts in long days. In an employee health screening, he learned that his cholesterol was 237 mg/dL. His doctor recommended that he go on a statin drug; however, because Erik was opposed to using a drug at that point, he came to the clinic looking for alternatives for reducing his high cholesterol. He wanted to try a more natural approach first.

When I asked him questions about his work life, it became clear that this was a big part of his problem. "I get to work around 7 A.M. and usually start my morning with a doughnut and coffee—the company provides them for free. I'm at my desk all morning, then I usually eat my lunch at my desk because I have too much work to do."

"What do you eat for lunch?" I asked him.

"Well, actually, someone usually goes to a local fast-food restaurant and gets lunch for all of us."

"How about dinner?"

"By the time I get off work around 9 P.M., I'm too tired to cook, so I pick up a sandwich or burger on my way home."

against heart disease than other alcoholic beverages. This connection has not been found in all studies, however.

Coffee?

Some observational studies have found an association between coffee intake and elevated cholesterol. However, because coffee use is typically associated with other bad habits, such as smoking and a diet high in animal fat, it is difficult to know for sure whether coffee is really causing the problem.[27]

It was apparent that Erik's job was interfering with his ability to get regular exercise and eat well. We talked about how he could fit exercise and eating better into his busy schedule, and he admitted that it was possible for him to take a lunch break if he wanted. He agreed to take a 15-minute walk around the grounds of his office and to bring his meals to work—including more fruits and vegetables in his lunches.

I saw Erik after 2 months, and his cholesterol had started to take a plunge. It had decreased from 237 mg/dL to 212 mg/dL. He said he was still eating quite a few burgers and fried foods, and he was going to cut back on those even more.

When I saw him after 1 more month, his cholesterol was down to a normal value of 193 mg/dL. He had virtually stopped his "burger run" after work, and he was eating more vegetables, fruits, and grains. It took him 3 months to make the necessary changes in his diet and lifestyle, but he never had to use a drug or supplement to control his cholesterol.

—Darin Ingels, N.D.

Changing Your Overall Lifestyle: It Really Does Work!

The bottom-line question for all of these lifestyle changes is, will they really reduce my risk of death or disease related to atherosclerosis? The answer is yes. It appears that a healthful lifestyle can not only lower your cholesterol but even reverse atherosclerosis.

The Lifestyle Heart Trial, a study spearheaded by Dr. Dean Ornish, demonstrated that lifestyle changes can reverse existing atherosclerosis.[28] This controlled study involved 48 participants with documented atherosclerosis in the arteries of their heart. Twenty-eight participants were randomly assigned to an experimental group that ate a lowfat vegetarian diet, stopped smoking, got moderate exercise, and underwent stress management training. The other 20 individuals were asked to continue living their normal life. These participants were followed for 1 year.

It appears that a healthful lifestyle can not only lower your cholesterol but even reverse atherosclerosis.

At the end of the year, each person was given an angiogram—a medical test that measures blockage in the arteries. Of the participants who made the lifestyle changes, 82% had less atherosclerosis than they had at the study's outset. The average blockage of the coronary arteries in the lifestyle change group dropped from 40 to 37.8%, while the blockage in the control group increased from 42.7 to 46%.

While it's difficult to say how much each separate lifestyle change contributed to the total effect, this study seems to demonstrate that exercising, choosing to eat a healthier diet, and avoiding high-risk activities may not only prevent—but actually reverse—atherosclerosis.

QUICK REVIEW

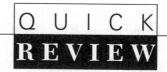

- A healthful lifestyle can lower cholesterol and possibly even reverse atherosclerosis.

- The single most important thing you can do to help prevent heart disease is to quit smoking.
- Eating a diet low in saturated fat and trans fatty acids may lower your cholesterol up to 25%, although 10 to 15% appears to be more common. Aim to reduce the total fat in your diet until it provides less than 30% of all the calories you consume.
- Other helpful changes include eating more fiber, while cutting down on meat and other animal-based foods (except cold-water fish).
- Regular aerobic exercise is important too; it can lower cholesterol by about 10 to 15%.
- The moderate use of alcohol, especially red wine, may have a beneficial effect on cholesterol.

Conventional Treatment for High Cholesterol

I f your cholesterol is high, it is important to lower it. If the natural treatments described in this book do not work, you need to take further steps. Conventional medications for high cholesterol (especially drugs in the statin family) are highly effective and produce few side effects.

How Effective Are Cholesterol-Lowering Drugs?

Very effective cholesterol-lowering drugs are available today. In clinical practice and in research, the statin drugs described in this chapter have been shown to lower total cholesterol by 25%, LDL ("bad") cholesterol by 35%, and triglycerides by 30%. They may also increase HDL ("good") cholesterol by 8%.

The first cholesterol-reducing "drug" was actually the vitamin niacin (vitamin B₃). It was introduced as a cholesterol-lowering agent more than 40 years ago, and it is still used today. As discussed in chapter 3, niacin has been shown to significantly improve cholesterol measurements, and it actually reduces mortality rates.

The first cholesterol-reducing "drug" was actually the vitamin niacin (vitamin B$_3$).

In the mid- to late 1960s, bile acid sequestering resins and fibric acid derivatives came on the market as alternatives to niacin. Bile acid sequestering drugs and fibric acid derivatives are fairly successful at lowering cholesterol, but have some problems that limit their clinical usefulness (more on these problems later in this chapter).

In 1987, the newest class of cholesterol-lowering drugs, the statin drugs, became available. As we will see, this class of drugs is more effective at lowering total cholesterol and LDL than the other drugs on the market, with substantially fewer side effects. We will discuss the statin drugs first, because they are the most widely used today. Then, we'll briefly discuss some of the older treatments.

The Statin Family: Powerful Medications with Few Side Effects

Statin drugs have greatly improved the treatment of high cholesterol. Drugs in this class include lovastatin (Mevacor), pravastatin (Pravachol), simvastatin (Zocor), fluvastatin (Lescol), and atorvastatin (Lipitor). They've been available in the United States for over 10 years, somewhat longer in European countries.

Lovastatin, the first of these drugs, was introduced in 1987. It was originally isolated from a strain of the common fungus *Aspergillus tereus*. Today, lovastatin is produced synthetically. Substances very similar to lovastatin are also found in red yeast rice (see chapter 4). Other statin drugs have subsequently been introduced by competing pharmaceutical companies. All of them appear to function similarly.

Statin drugs work by interfering with the body's normal production of cholesterol. In the liver and other tissues, an enzyme called HMG-CoA reductase controls the rate at which the body manufactures cholesterol. When your cholesterol level is low, your body produces more HMG-CoA reductase, which in turn creates more cholesterol. When your cholesterol levels are where they should be, HMG-CoA production is turned off. In this way, your body has a built-in mechanism, like a thermostat, to keep cholesterol levels in the

Statin drugs are more effective at lowering total cholesterol and LDL than the other drugs on the market, with substantially fewer side effects.

optimal range, neither too high nor too low. When your cholesterol levels are too high it is because this built-in function is not working properly.

The statin drugs directly affect the body's "thermostat" by inhibiting the action of HMG-CoA reductase. (Interestingly, garlic may work the same way, and red yeast rice almost certainly does. See chapters 2 and 4 for more about these treatments.) When you take a drug or herb that inhibits HMG-CoA reductase, you inhibit the body's ability to produce more cholesterol. The net result is that cholesterol levels decline.

Of all the cholesterol-lowering drugs, this class is by far the most effective. The Scandinavian Simvastatin Survival

Sam's Story

Sam was a 37-year-old athlete. "It's not fair," he told me the first time we met. "I exercise 2 hours daily and run marathons. I'm also a vegetarian, and the only fat I get is from olive oil and canola oil. Yet my total cholesterol level is over 375. Why is the universe picking on me?"

It turned out that Sam's father had died of a heart attack at age 47. This event was partly responsible for Sam's vigorous lifestyle: He didn't want the same thing to happen to him. "Only nothing I do seems to be working," he complained.

Clearly, for Sam there was a genetic factor at work. It was probably genetics that killed his father, and the same would happen to him if he didn't successfully lower his cholesterol.

Study, published in 1995, was a double-blind placebo-controlled trial that evaluated 4,444 participants with a history of either chest pain or previous heart attack.[1] Half the group received simvastatin while the other half received placebo that looked just like the drug. Researchers followed both groups for just over 5 years.

Statin drugs work by interfering with the body's normal production of cholesterol.

This study showed just how effective statin drugs really are. Total cholesterol fell by 25%, and LDL cholesterol dropped 35% while HDL cholesterol went up 8%. Furthermore, this study added a very important finding: There was a whopping 42% decrease in death from heart disease in the group taking simvastatin, and a 30% de

I reassured Sam that his lifestyle was helping him. "Even if it isn't lowering your cholesterol, it is undoubtedly adding to your life span," I told him. "But you need to take other steps, too."

I did not suggest that he try any herbs or supplements. His cholesterol was simply too high. On my suggestion, he took the cholesterol-lowering drug simvastatin, and within 2 months his total cholesterol was under 200. This tremendous improvement was a testament not only to the medication, but also to Sam's lifestyle. He had done his part; adding a medication carried him the rest of the way.

—Steven Bratman, M.D.

crease in death from all causes. While 12% of the participants in the placebo group died during the course of the study, only 8% of the people in the simvastatin group died. Thus, this study showed that taking a statin drug can increase long-term survival.

This type of study is important because it shows that the drug is doing what we want it to do. Although we know that high cholesterol is associated with increased death from heart disease, this does not guarantee that a drug that lowers cholesterol will actually reduce the risk of death from heart disease. Drugs have many effects, and it is always possible that unrecognized bad effects may outweigh the good ones. This study showed that simvastatin produces an effect that is highly beneficial overall.

Nearly identical results were seen in similar studies of pravastatin and lovastatin.[2,3]

All of the statin drugs are effective at lowering cholesterol. However, as with most classes of medications, people react to the statin drugs in individual ways. For example, a person who may not see any cholesterol reduction with lovastatin can be switched to pravastatin or simvastatin and see substantial results. It is not clear why this phenomenon occurs, but it is typical of all medical treatments, including herbs. (A new area of drug research, called *pharmacogenetics,* is beginning to help us understand why this may be. It appears that different responses to drugs can sometimes be accounted for by genetic differences in the people taking the drugs.)

Safety Issues

Besides their effectiveness, another major advantage to statin drugs is that they have a low incidence of side effects. The most common problem is headache, but it occurs in less than 2% of those who take these medications. Also, a small number of people have allergic reactions to these drugs. Other occasional side effects of statin drugs include abdominal pain, constipation, diarrhea, nausea, dizziness, skin rash, blurred vision, and joint pain; however, these side effects go away when you stop taking the drug.

There were some early reports that these drugs caused opacification, or clouding of the lens in the eye. But larger studies have since found that this is not true. However, there are some significant safety concerns when using these medications: liver toxicity, muscle and kidney damage, possible cancer risk, and CoQ_{10} depletion.

Liver Toxicity

A serious potential side effect of statin drugs is liver toxicity. In studies, about 1 to 2% of those who take these drugs show signs of significant liver inflammation. Physicians evaluate the health of the liver by measuring the level of enzymes that normally leak out of the liver. When the liver cells become damaged, these enzymes leak out at an increased rate, raising levels of these enzymes in the blood. For this reason, you will hear the description "elevated liver enzymes" to describe evidence of liver problems.

In one large study of pravastatin, about 1% of the treated group showed a threefold elevation in liver enzymes.[4] This is not as bad as it sounds, however, because there was a similar elevation in 0.75% of the placebo group, showing that, in many cases, the elevation of enzymes was due to something other than the treatment. For example, even modest use of alcohol elevates liver enzymes. Still, your liver is so important that current recommendations suggest that if you take a statin drug, you need to check your liver enzymes after 6 weeks of therapy. Fortunately, liver enzymes generally return to normal soon after the drug is stopped.

Muscle and Kidney Damage

A rare but very serious side effect of statin drugs is an inflammation of the muscles that causes severe muscle damage. Even worse, the products of dying muscle can destroy the kidney. This rare and little understood side effect has mostly been seen when statin drugs are combined with certain other medications, such as niacin, erythromycin, cyclosporine, or fibrate drugs. Your physician or pharmacist can advise you whether it is safe to combine statins with other medications you may be taking.

Do Statin Drugs Increase Cancer Risk?

Probably the biggest question regarding statin drugs is lingering concerns that they may increase the risk of cancer. Laboratory tests on mice have found a slight but significant increase in the incidence of certain cancers in female mice (but not in male mice). Other studies have found an increased cancer incidence in both male and female rodents at doses 3 to 33 times higher than the usual human dose, and still other animal studies have found that HMG-CoA reductase inhibitors cause mutation in cells, the usual first step in the development of cancer.

None of the studies on humans have found a significantly increased incidence of cancer; however, these studies did not run the 20 or 30 years that would be necessary to discover long-term risks.

Some respected medical authorities have interpreted the animal research findings to mean that the statin drugs should not even be on the market. Others point to the dramatic evidence of reduction in death from heart disease, and feel that the benefits outweigh the risk.

There is no simple answer to this controversy. Many of these issues can only be answered over time with careful examination of the magnitude of the risks and benefits of using these drugs. We recommend that you consult closely with your physician to decide whether these medications are appropriate for you.

Coenzyme Q_{10} Depletion

An important but rarely recognized side effect of taking a statin drug is the depletion of a naturally occurring substance called coenzyme Q_{10} (CoQ_{10}).[5,6] It appears that the very same process that inhibits HMG-CoA reductase also reduces CoQ_{10} production. This side effect is "silent," because there are no obvious symptoms that occur when CoQ_{10} levels drop. It's not entirely clear whether CoQ_{10} depletion causes any health problems, but the result probably isn't that great for you.

CoQ_{10} is a nutrient that we need to transform food into energy. It is found in almost every cell of the body. CoQ_{10} is also a powerful antioxidant. CoQ_{10} can be taken as a supplement, and it has been used to treat a variety of health conditions, especially those related to heart disease.

Although we don't know for sure what the consequences of CoQ_{10} depletion may be, it may be wise to take 30 mg daily as insurance. CoQ_{10} appears to be a very safe supplement. The maximum safe dosage in young children, pregnant or nursing women, or those with severe liver or kidney disease has not been determined. (For more information on CoQ_{10}, see *The Natural Pharmacist: Your Complete Guide to Vitamins and Supplements*.)

Bile Acid Sequestering Resins: Too Many Side Effects

Cholestyramine (Questran) and colestipol (Colestid) are members of one of the oldest categories of drugs used to lower cholesterol, the bile acid sequestering resins. Although effective, these drugs have fallen out of favor because of their relatively high incidence of side effects. Cholestyramine and colestipol work in an interesting, roundabout away.

Bile acids are formed in the liver and used to break down fatty foods. They contain considerable quantities of cholesterol. Normally, after bile acids have done their work on a fatty meal, the body reabsorbs them and the cholesterol they contain. Bile acid sequestering resins work by binding to numerous substances, including bile acids. As these drugs move

Although effective, bile acid sequestering resins have fallen out of favor because of their relatively high incidence of side effects.

through the intestinal tract, they act like a strong magnet attracting bile acids and forming a combined molecule that cannot be reabsorbed. This cholesterol is then lost to the body.

In order to make more bile acids, the liver has to get some spare cholesterol from somewhere. One of its main sources is cholesterol floating about in the blood. The net result of this complex chain of events is that cholesterol levels in the blood are reduced.

These drugs typically reduce total cholesterol by about 10%, and decrease LDL cholesterol by up to 20%, while raising HDL cholesterol by 3 to 8%.

Unfortunately, bile acid sequestering resins pose several problems. They are taken in the form of powder, which is mixed with liquid and drunk like a milkshake. This "resin milkshake" tastes terrible to most people. One man described his experience as "trying to drink sand in rotten milk." Some people try to mix the powder in juice or applesauce to mask the taste and texture, but you won't find too many people rushing to the pharmacy to fill this prescription as a taste treat.

Another problem is gastrointestinal side effects such as bloating, diarrhea, flatulence, nausea, vomiting, and constipation. While not dangerous, these side effects can be extremely unpleasant. Furthermore, along with cholesterol, these resins also remove fat-soluble vitamins from the body, such as vitamins A, D, E, and K. If they are used for a long period of time, genuine deficiencies might develop. One of the most serious possible consequences is an excess tendency to bleed due to vitamin K deficiency.

Resins can also bind a variety of medications that we'd rather keep within our bodies, such as penicillin, digoxin (a heart medication), propranolol (taken for high blood pressure), thyroid hormone, and warfarin (taken to prevent blood clotting). People using resin drugs are advised to take any other medication at least 1 hour before or 4 hours after taking the resin.

Fibric Acid Derivatives:
Better for Treating High Triglyceride Levels

Triglycerides can also increase the risk of heart disease, although they are not as dangerous as cholesterol. Still, if triglyceride levels are high enough, they can cause problems. The fibric acid drugs are most useful for people with mildly elevated cholesterol but very high triglyceride levels.

This class of drugs includes gemfibrozil (Lopid) and clofibrate (Atromid-S). We do not really know how they work. However, there is no question that they do work. A 5-year double-blind placebo-controlled study of 4,081 men found that gemfibrozil reduced triglycerides by 35%, but only reduced

The fibric acid drugs are most useful for people with mildly elevated cholesterol but very high triglyceride levels.

cholesterol by 8%. Over this 5-year period, there was an overall decrease of 34% in mortality from coronary heart disease.[7]

However, other studies have not shown any reduction in death from cardiovascular disease, and a few have even shown an overall *increase* as high as 44% in the rate of death due to conditions other than cardiovascular diseases, including cancer, complications following gallbladder removal, and pancreatitis (inflammation of the pancreas).[8]

Fibric acid drugs also cause significant digestive upset in as many as 34% of people who take them.[9] Rarer but more severe side effects include gallbladder disease, liver inflammation, muscle inflammation, kidney damage, and bone marrow injury. Finally, there is a concern that these drugs may increase the incidence of cancer.

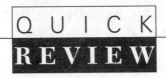

QUICK REVIEW

- The leading treatments today are the statin drugs. This class of medications is significantly more effective and causes fewer side effects than the other conventional medications for reducing cholesterol.

- An important 5-year study found that statin drugs can significantly reduce the incidence of death from heart disease.

- Statin drugs can cause liver inflammation.

- Other types of cholesterol-reducing medications include the bile acid sequestering resins and fibric acid derivatives. However, they are less effective, have more side effects, and are used less frequently. Fibric acid drugs are most useful for people with very high triglyceride levels.

Putting It
All Together

or your easy reference, this chapter contains a
brief summary of key information on treatments
described in this book. Please refer to earlier
chapters for more comprehensive information, including a
detailed discussion of dosage and safety issues.

Natural Treatments for Lowering Cholesterol

Garlic appears to have only a modest effect on reducing
cholesterol, but it also offers other heart-healthy benefits
that combine and promote overall heart health.

High-dose **niacin** is quite effective at reducing bad
cholesterol and raising good cholesterol. However, it can
cause flushing as well as liver inflammation. This supplement should not be combined with statin drugs except
under close physician supervision.

Stanol esters, added to some supermarket margarines, are thought to work by interfering with the body's
ability to manufacture cholesterol. If you are already

taking statin drugs, stanol esters can improve your cholesterol levels even more.

The supplement **policosanol** appears to improve cholesterol levels, and it too may offer added benefits if combined with statin drugs.

Soy foods also lower cholesterol levels, as well as providing other important health benefits.

Red yeast rice is a natural source of chemicals in the statin drug family, and it may help decrease total and LDL cholesterol levels.

One double-blind study suggests that **artichoke leaf** may reduce cholesterol levels.

Other treatments with some evidence of effectiveness include **guggul, pantethine, tocotrienols, fish oil,** and **carnitine,** and to a lesser extent creatine, calcium, probiotics and spirulina.

Natural Treatments for Cholesterol-Related Side Effects of Drugs

Medications in the beta-blocker family sometimes reduce levels of HDL cholesterol. The supplement **chromium** may help counter this.

Another positive interaction with a medication involves a combination of **vitamins C** and **E** and the drug tamoxifen. Tamoxifen has a tendency to raise triglyceride levels. One study found that vitamin C and vitamin E together may counteract this side effect.

Lifestyle Changes

Diet and lifestyle can reduce cholesterol levels, reverse atherosclerosis, and protect you from a variety of illnesses and health risks. If you want to reduce your risk of heart disease, the single most important change you can make in your lifestyle is to quit smoking. A diet low in saturated (animal) fats and trans fatty acids (margarine), and high in polyunsaturated and monounsaturated fats, can significantly reduce your cholesterol level. Eating more nuts and adding more fiber to your diet may also be useful.

A regular aerobic exercise program can also help improve your cholesterol levels and your overall health.

However, if your cholesterol levels remain high despite the natural approaches we've presented, you will need to take further steps. Medications in the statin family are highly effective, and generally produce few side effects.

Notes

Chapter 1: Atherosclerosis and High Cholesterol

1. Robbins S, Cotran R, Kumar V. *Robbins Pathologic Basis of Disease*. 5th ed. Philadelphia, Pa: Saunders; 1994.

2. Strong JP, Malcom CT, Newman WP III, et al. Early lesions of atherosclerosis in childhood and youth: natural history and risk factors. *J Am Coll Nutr*. 1992;11:51S–54S.

3. Strong JP. The natural history of atherosclerosis in childhood. *Ann N Y Acad Sci*. 1991;623:9–15.

4. Schaefer EJ, Lamon-Fava S, Jenner JL, et al. Lipoprotein(a) levels and risk of coronary heart disease in men. The Lipid Research Clinics Coronary Primary Prevention Trial. *JAMA*. 1994;271:999–1003.

5. Scanu AM. Lipoprotein(a). A genetic risk factor for premature coronary heart disease. *JAMA*. 1992;267:3326–3329.

Chapter 2: Garlic and High Cholesterol

1. Mader FH. Treatment of hyperlipidaemia with garlic-powder tablets. Evidence from the German Association of General Practitioners' multicentric placebo-controlled double-blind study. *Arzneimittelforschung*. 1990;40: 1111–1116.

2. Greenberg RP, Bornstein RF, Zborowski MJ, et al. A meta-analysis of fluoxetine outcome in the treatment of depression. *J Nerv Ment Dis*. 1994;182:547–551.

3. Jain AK, Vargas R, Gotzkowsky S, et al. Can garlic reduce levels of serum lipids? A controlled clinical study. *Am J Med*. 1993;94:632–635.

4. Holzgartner H, Schmidt U, Kuhn U. Comparison of the efficacy and tolerance of a garlic preparation vs. bezafibrate. *Arzneimittelforschung.* 1992;42:1473–1477.

5. Steiner M, Khsan AH, Holbert D, et al. A double-blind crossover study in moderately hypercholesterolemic men that compared the effect of aged garlic extract and placebo administration on blood lipids. *Am J Clin Nutr.* 1996;64: 866–870.

6. Neil HA, Silagy CA, Lancaster T, et al. Garlic powder in the treatment of moderate hyperlipidaemia: a controlled trial and meta-analysis. *J R Coll Physicians Lond.* 1996;30: 329–334.

7. Simons LA, Balasubramaniam S, von Konigsmark M, et al. On the effect of garlic on plasma lipids and lipoproteins in mild hypercholesterolaemia. *Atherosclerosis.* 1995;113: 219–225.

8. Superko HR, Krauss RM. Garlic powder, effect on plasma lipids, postprandial lipemia, low-density lipoprotein particle size, high-density lipoprotein subclass distribution and lipoprotein(a). *J Am Coll Cardiol.* 2000;35:321–326.

9. Isaacsohn JL, Moser M, Stein EA, et al. Garlic powder and plasma lipids and lipoproteins: a multicenter, randomized, placebo-controlled trial. *Arch Intern Med.* 1998;158: 1189–1194.

10. Stevinson C. Pittler MH, Ernst E. Garlic for treating hypercholesterolemia. A meta-analysis of randomized clinical trials. *Ann Intern Med.* 2000;133:420–429.

11. Stevinson C, Pittler MH, Ernst E. Garlic for treating hypercholesterolemia. A meta-analysis of randomized clinical trials. *Ann Intern Med.* 2000;133:420–429.

12. Lachmann G, Lorenz D, Radeck W, et al. The pharmacokinetics of the S35 labeled garlic constituents alliin, allicin and vinyldithiine [in German; English abstract]. *Arzneimittelforschung.* 1994;44:734–743.

13. Qureshi AA, Abuirmeileh N, Din ZZ, et al. Inhibition of cholesterol and fatty acid biosynthesis in liver enzymes and chicken hepatocytes by polar fractions of garlic. *Lipids.* 1983;18:343–348.

14. Gebhardt, R. Multiple inhibitory effects of garlic extracts on cholesterol biosynthesis in hepatocytes. *Lipids.* 1993;28: 613–619.

15. Gebhardt R, Beck H. Differential inhibitory effects of garlic-derived organosulfur compounds on cholesterol biosynthesis in primary rat hepatocyte cultures. *Lipids.* 1996;31: 1269–1276.

16. Yeh YY, Yeh SM. Garlic reduces plasma lipids by inhibiting hepatic cholesterol and triacylglycerol synthesis. *Lipids.* 1994;29:189–193.

17. Sendl A, Schliack M, Loser R, et al. Inhibition of cholesterol synthesis in vitro by extracts and isolated compounds prepared from garlic and wild garlic. *Atherosclerosis.* 1992;94:79–85.

18. Gebhardt R, Beck H. Differential inhibitory effects of garlic-derived organosulfur compounds on cholesterol biosynthesis in primary rat hepatocyte cultures. *Lipids.* 1996; 31:1269–1276.

19. Eilat S, Oestraicher Y, Rabinkov A, et al. Alteration of lipid profile in hyperlipidemic rabbits by allicin, an active constituent of garlic. *Coron Artery Dis.* 1995;6:985–990.

20. Chandorkar AG, Jain PK. Analysis of hypotensive action of *Allium sativum* (garlic) [abstract]. *Indian J Physiol Pharmacol.* 1973;17:132–133.

21. Foushee DB, Ruffin J, Banerjee U. Garlic as a natural agent for the treatment of hypertension: a preliminary report. *Cytobios.* 1982;34:145–152.

22. Auer W, Eiber A, Hertkorn E, et al. Hypertension and hyperlipidaemia: garlic helps in mild cases. *Br J Clin Pract Suppl.* 1990;69: 3–6.

23. Silagy CA, Neil HA. A meta-analysis of the effect of garlic on blood pressure. *J Hypertens.* 1994;12:463–468.

24. Das I, Khan NS, Sooranna SR. Potent activation of nitric oxide synthase by garlic: a basis for its therapeutic applications. *Curr Med Res Opin.* 1995;13:257–263.

25. Pedraza-Chaverri J, Tapia E, Medina-Campos ON, et al. Garlic prevents hypertension induced by chronic inhibition of nitric oxide synthesis. *Life Sci.* 1998;62:PL 71–77.

26. Dirsch VM, Kiemer AK, Wagner H, et al. Effect of allicin and ajoene, two compounds of garlic, on inducible nitric oxide synthase. *Atherosclerosis*. 1998;139:333–339.

27. Siegel G, Emden J, Wenzel K, et al. Potassium channel activation in vascular smooth muscle. *Adv Exp Med Biol*. 1992; 311:53–72.

28. Siegel G, Walter A, Schnalke F, et al. Potassium channel activation, hyperpolarization, and vascular relaxation. *Z Kardiol*. 1991;80(suppl 7):9–24.

29. Orekhov AN, Grunwald J. Effects of garlic on atherosclerosis. *Nutrition*. 1997;13:656–663.

30. Breithaupt-Grogler K, Ling M, Boudoulas H, et al. Protective effect of chronic garlic intake on elastic properties of aorta in the elderly. *Circulation*. 1997;96:2649–2655.

31. Das I, Khan NS, Sooranna SR. Potent activation of nitric oxide synthase by garlic: a basis for its therapeutic applications. *Curr Med Res Opin*. 1995;13:257–263.

32. Steiner M, Lin RS. Changes in platelet function and susceptibility of lipoproteins to oxidation associated with administration of aged garlic extract. *J Cardiovasc Pharmacol*. 1998;31:904–908.

33. Kiesewetter H, Jung F, Pindur G, et al. Effect of garlic on thrombocyte aggregation, microcirculation, and other risk factors. *Int J Clin Pharmacol Ther Toxicol*. 1991;29: 151–155.

34. Kleijnen J, Knipschild P, ter Reit G. Garlic, onions and cardiovascular risk factors. A review of the evidence from human experiments with emphasis on commercially available preparations. *Br J Clin Pharmacol*. 1989;28:535–544.

35. Reuter HD. *Allium sativum* and *Allium ursinum*: part 2 pharmacology and medicinal application. *Phytomedicine*. 1995;2:73–91.

36. Reuter HD, Sendl A. *Allium sativum* and *Allium ursinum*: chemistry, pharmacology and medical applications. *Econ Med Plant Res*. 1994;6:55–113.

37. Chutani SK, Bordia A. The effect of fried versus raw garlic on fibrinolytic activity in man. *Atherosclerosis*. 1981;38: 417–421.

38. Yamasaki T, Lau BH. Garlic compounds protect vascular endothelial cells from oxidant injury. *Nippon Yakurigaku Zasshi.* 1997;110:138–141.

39. Lewin G, Popov I. Antioxidant effects of aqueous garlic extract. 2nd communication: inhibition of the Cu(2+)-initiated oxidation of low density lipoproteins. *Arzneimittelforschung.* 1994;44:604–607.

40. Ide N, Lau BH. Garlic compounds protect vascular endothelial cells from oxidized low density lipoprotein-induced injury. *J Pharm Pharmacol.* 1997;49:908–911.

41. Horie T, Awazu S, Itakura Y, et al. Identified diallyl polysulfides from an aged garlic extract which protects the membranes from lipid peroxidation. *Planta Med.* 1992;58:468–469.

42. Phelps S, Harris WS. Garlic supplementation and lipoprotein oxidation susceptibility. *Lipids.* 1993;28:475–477.

43. Prasad K, Laxdal VA, Yu M, et al. Antioxidant activity of allicin, an active principle in garlic. *Mol Cell Biochem.* 1995;148:183–189.

44. Imai J, Ide N, Nagae S, et al. Antioxidant and radical scavenging effects of aged garlic extract and its constituents. *Planta Med.* 1994;60:417–420.

45. Yamasaki T, Lau BH. Garlic compounds protect vascular endothelial cells from oxidant injury. *Nippon Yakurigaku Zasshi.* 1997;110:138–141.

46. Koscielny J, Klussendorf D, Latza R, et al. The antiatherosclerotic effect of *Allium sativum. Atherosclerosis.* 1999;144:237–249.

47. Bordia A. Garlic and coronary heart disease [translated from German]. *Dtsch Apoth Ztg.* 1989;129:16–17.

48. Fleischauer AT, Poole C, Arab L. Garlic consumption and cancer prevention: meta-analyses of colorectal and stomach cancers. *Am J Clin Nutr.* 2000;72:1047–1052.

49. Agarwal KC. Therapeutic actions of garlic constituents. *Med Res Rev.* 1996;16:111–124.

50. Dausch JG, Nixon DW. Garlic: a review of its relationship to malignant disease. *Prev Med.* 1990;19:346–361.

51. Dorant E, van den Brandt PA, Goldbohm RA, et al. Garlic and its significance for the prevention of cancer in humans: a critical view. *Br J Cancer.* 1993;67:424–429.

52. Lau BH, Tadi PP, Tosk JM. *Allium sativum* (garlic) and cancer prevention. *Nutr Res.* 1990;10:937–948.

53. Steinmetz KA, Kushi LH, Bostick RM, et al. Vegetables, fruit, and colon cancer in the Iowa Women's Health Study. *Am J Epidemiol.* 1994;139:1–15.

54. You WC, Blot WJ, Chang YS, et al. *Allium* vegetables and reduced risk of stomach cancer. *J Natl Cancer Inst.* 1989; 81:162–164.

55. Ernst E. Can *Allium* vegetables prevent cancer? *Phytomedicine.* 1997;4:79–83.

56. Schulz V, Hansel R, Tyler VE. *Rational Phytotherapy: A Physicians' Guide to Herbal Medicine.* 3rd ed. Berlin, Germany: Springer-Verlag; 1998: 121–122.

57. Mader FH. Treatment of hyperlipidaemia with garlic-powder tablets. Evidence from the German Association of General Practitioners' multicentric placebo-controlled double-blind study. *Arzneimittelforschung.* 1990;40:1111–1116.

58. Schulz V, Hansel R, Tyler VE. *Rational Phytotherapy: A Physicians' Guide to Herbal Medicine.* 3rd ed. Berlin, Germany: Springer-Verlag; 1998.

59. Burden AD, Wilkinson SM, Beck MH, et al. Garlic-induced systemic contact dermatitis. *Contact Dermatitis.* 1994;30: 299–300.

60. McFadden JP, White IR, Rycroft RJ. Allergic contact dermatitis from garlic. *Contact Dermatitis.* 1992;27:333–334.

61. Lembo G, Balato N, Patruno C, et al. Allergic contact dermatitis due to garlic *(Allium sativum). Contact Dermatitis.* 1991;25:330–331.

62. Sumiyoshi H, Kanezawa A, Masamoto K, et al. Chronic toxicity test of garlic extract in rats [in Japanese; English abstract]. *J Toxicol Sci.* 1984;9:61–75.

63. Yoshida S, Hirao Y, Nakagawa S. Mutagenicity and cytotoxicity tests of garlic [in Japanese; English abstract]. *J Toxicol Sci.* 1984;9:77–86.

64. German K, Kumar U, Blackford HN. Garlic and the risk of TURP bleeding. *Br J Urol.* 1995;76:518.

65. Burnham BE. Garlic as a possible risk for postoperative bleeding. *Plast Reconstr Surg.* 1995;95:213.

66. Piscitelli SC. Use of complementary medicines by patients with HIV: Full sail into uncharted waters. *Medscape HIV/AIDS.* 2000;6.

67. Abdullah TH, Kirkpatrick DV, Carter J. Enhancement of natural killer cell activity in AIDS with garlic. *Dtsch Zschr Onkol.* 1989;21:52–53.

68. Kandil OM, Abdullah TH, Elkadi A. Garlic and the immune system in humans: its effects on natural killer cells [abstract]. *Fed Proc.* 1987;46:441.

69. Fleischauer AT, Poole C, Arab L. Garlic consumption and cancer prevention: meta-analyses of colorectal and stomach cancers. *Am J Clin Nutr.* 2000;72:1047–1052.

Chapter 3: Niacin and High Cholesterol

1. Canner PL, Berge KG, Wenger NK, et al. Fifteen year mortality in Coronary Drug Project patients: long term benefit with niacin. *J Am Coll Cardiol.* 1986;8:1245–1255.

2. McKenney JM, Proctor JD, Harris S, et al. A comparison of the efficacy and toxic effects of sustained- vs. immediate-release niacin in hypercholesterolemic patients. *JAMA.* 1994;271:672–677.

3. Christensen NA, Achor RW, Berge KG, et al. Nicotinic acid treatment of hypercholesteremia. *JAMA.* 1961;177:546–550.

4. Knopp RH, Ginsberg J, Albers JJ, et al. Contrasting effects of unmodified and time-release forms of niacin on lipoproteins in hyperlipidemic subjects: clues to mechanism of action of niacin. *Metabolism.* 1995;34:642–650.

5. Superko HR, Krauss RM. Differential effects of nicotinic acid in subjects with different LDL subclass patterns. *Atherosclerosis.* 1992;95:69–76.

6. Elam MB, Hunninghake DB, Davis KB, et al. Effect of niacin on lipid and lipoprotein levels and glycemic control in patients with diabetes and peripheral arterial disease:

the ADMIT study. A randomized trial. Arterial Disease Multiple Intervention Trial. *JAMA*. 2000;284:1263–1270.

7. Morgan JM, Capuzzi DM, Guyton JR, et al. Treatment effect of Niaspan™, a controlled-release niacin, in patients with hypercholesterolemia: a placebo-controlled trial. *J Cardiovasc Pharmacol Ther*. 1996;1:195–202.

8. Guyton JR, Goldberg AC, Kreisberg RA, et al. Effectiveness of once-nightly dosing of extended-release niacin alone and in combination for hypercholesterolemia. *Am J Cardiol*. 1998;82:737–743.

9. Illingworth DR, Stein EA, Mitchel YB, et al. Comparative effects of lovastatin and niacin in primary hypercholesterolemia. A prospective trial. *Arch Intern Med*. 1994;154: 1586–1595.

10. Smith CM, Reynard AM, eds. *Essentials of Pharmacology*. Philadelphia, Pa: W.B. Saunders; 1995: 306.

11. Alderman JD, Pasternak RC, Sacks FM, et al. Effect of a modified, well-tolerated niacin regimen on serum total cholesterol, high density lipoprotein cholesterol and the cholesterol to high density lipoprotein ratio. *Am J Cardiol*. 1989;64:725–729.

12. Jungnickel PW, Maloley PA, Tuin ELV, et al. Effect of two aspirin pretreatment regimens on niacin-induced cutaneous reactions. *J Gen Intern Med*. 1997;12:591–596.

13. Head KA. Inositol hexaniacinate: A safer alternative to niacin. *Alt Med Rev*. 1996;1:176–184.

14. McKenney JM, Proctor JD, Harris S, et al. A comparison of the efficacy and toxic effects of sustained- vs immediate-release niacin in hypercholesterolemic patients. *JAMA*. 1994;271:672–677.

15. Guyton JR, Goldberg AC, Kreisberg RA, et al. Effectiveness of once-nightly dosing of extended-release niacin alone and in combination for hypercholesterolemia. *Am J Cardiol*. 1998;82:737–743.

16. Head KA. Inositol hexaniacinate: A safer alternative to niacin. *Alt Med Rev*. 1996;1:176–184.

17. Clementz GL, Holmes AW. Nicotinic acid-induced fulminant hepatic failure. *J Clin Gastroenterol*. 1987;9:582–584.

18. Guyton JR, Goldberg AC, Kreisberg RA, et al. Effectiveness of once-nightly dosing of extended-release niacin alone and in combination for hypercholesterolemia. *Am J Cardiol*. 1998;82:737–743.

19. Jacobsen TA, Amorosa LF. Combination therapy with fluvastatin and niacin in hypercholesterolemia: a preliminary report on safety. *Am J Cardiol*. 1994;73:25D–29D.

20. Elam MB, Hunninghake DB, Davis KB, et al. Effect of niacin on lipid and lipoprotein levels and glycemic control in patients with diabetes and peripheral arterial disease: the ADMIT study. A randomized trial. Arterial Disease Multiple Intervention Trial. *JAMA*. 2000;284:1263–1270.

21. *Physicians' Desk Reference for Nonprescription Drugs and Dietary Supplements*. Montvale, NJ: Medical Economics Co; 1999: 1507.

22. Colletti RB, Neufeld EJ, Roff NK, et al. Niacin treatment of hypercholesterolemia in children. *Pediatrics*. 1993;92: 78–82.

Chapter 4: Other Evidence-Based Natural Treatments for High Cholesterol

1. Nguyen TT. The cholesterol-lowering action of plant stanol esters. *J Nutr*. 1999;129:2109–2112.

2. Gylling H, Miettinen TA. Cholesterol reduction by different plant stanol mixtures and with variable fat intake. *Metabolism*. 1999;48:575–580.

3. Blair SN, Capuzzi DM, Gottlieb SO, et al. Incremental reduction of serum total cholesterol and low-density lipoprotein cholesterol with the addition of plant stanol ester-containing spread to statin therapy. *Am J Cardiol*. 2000;86:46–52.

4. Tammi A, Ronnemaa T, Gylling H, et al. Plant stanol ester margarine lowers serum total and low-density lipoprotein cholesterol concentrations of healthy children: the STRIP project. Special Turku Coronary Risk Factors Intervention Project. *J Pediatr*. 2000;136:503–510.

5. Law M. Plant sterol and stanol margarines and health. *BMJ*. 2000;320:861–864.

6. Gylling H, Miettinen TA. Serum cholesterol and cholesterol and lipoprotein metabolism in hypercholesterolaemic
NIDDM patients before and during sitostanol ester-
margarine treatment. *Diabetologia*. 1994;37:773–780.

7. Gylling H, Miettinen TA. Cholesterol reduction by different plant stanol mixtures and with variable fat intake. *Metabolism*. 1999;48:575–580.

8. Vanhanen HT, Blomqvist S, Ehnholm C, et al. Serum cholesterol, cholesterol precursors, and plant sterols in hypercholesterolemic subjects with different apoE phenotypes
during dietary sitostanol ester treatment. *J Lipid Res*.
1993;34:1535–1544.

9. Blair SN, Capuzzi DM, Gottlieb SO, et al. Incremental reduction of serum total cholesterol and low-density lipoprotein cholesterol with the addition of plant stanol
ester-containing spread to statin therapy. *Am J Cardiol*.
2000;86:46–52.

10. Nguyen TT, Dale LV, von Bergmann K, et al. Cholesterol-
lowering effect of stanol ester in a US population of mildly
hypercholesterolemic men and women: a randomized controlled trial. *Mayo Clin Proc*. 1999;74:1198–2206.

11. Miettinen TA, Puska P, Gylling H, et al. Reduction of
serum cholesterol with sitostanol-ester margarine in a
mildly hypercholesterolemic population. *N Engl J Med*.
1995;333:1308–1312.

12. Hallikainen MA, Sarkkinen ES, Uusitupa MI. Effects of
low-fat stanol ester enriched margarines on concentrations
of serum carotenoids in subjects with elevated serum cholesterol concentrations. *Eur J Clin Nutr*. 1999;53:966–969.

13. Gylling H, Siimes MA, Miettinen TA. Sitostanol ester margarine in dietary treatment of children with familial hypercholesterolemia. *J Lipid Res*. 1995;36:1807–1812.

14. Tammi A, Ronnemaa T, Gylling H, et al. Plant stanol ester
margarine lowers serum total and low-density lipoprotein
cholesterol concentrations of healthy children: the STRIP
project. Special Turku Coronary Risk Factors Intervention
Project. *J Pediatr*. 2000;136:503–510.

15. Hallikainen MA, Uusitupa MI. Effects of 2 low-fat stanol
ester-containing margarines on serum cholesterol concen-

trations as part of a low-fat diet in hypercholesterolemic subjects. *Am J Clin Nutr*. 1999;69:403–410.

16. Gylling H, Radhakrishnan R, Miettinen TA. Reduction of serum cholesterol in postmenopausal women with previous myocardial infarction and cholesterol malabsorption induced by dietary sitostanol ester margarine: women and dietary sitostanol. *Circulation*. 1997;96:4226–4231.

17. Jones PJ, Ntanios FY, Raeini-Sarjaz M, et al. Cholesterol-lowering efficacy of a sitostanol-containing phytosterol mixture with a prudent diet in hyperlipidemic men. *Am J Clin Nutr*. 1999;69:1144–1150.

18. Vanhanen HT, Kajander J, Lehtovirta H, et al. Serum levels, absorption efficiency, faecal elimination and synthesis of cholesterol during increasing doses of dietary sitostanol esters in hypercholesterolaemic subjects. *Clin Sci (Colch)*. 1994;87:61–67.

19. Nguyen TT. The cholesterol-lowering action of plant stanol esters. *J Nutr*. 1999;129:2109–2112.

20. Miettinen TA, Puska P, Gylling H, et al. Reduction of serum cholesterol with sitostanol-ester margarine in a mildly hypercholesterolemic population. *N Engl J Med*. 1995;333: 1308–1312.

21. Gylling H, Miettinen TA. Effects of inhibiting cholesterol absorption and synthesis on cholesterol and lipoprotein metabolism in hypercholesterolemic non-insulin-dependent diabetic men. *J Lipid Res*. 1996;37:1776–1785.

22. Blair SN, Capuzzi DM, Gottlieb SO, et al. Incremental reduction of serum total cholesterol and low-density lipoprotein cholesterol with the addition of plant stanol ester-containing spread to statin therapy. *Am J Cardiol*. 2000;86:46–52.

23. Blair SN, Capuzzi DM, Gottlieb SO, et al. Incremental reduction of serum total cholesterol and low-density lipoprotein cholesterol with the addition of plant stanol ester-containing spread to statin therapy. *Am J Cardiol*. 2000;86:46–52.

24. Miettinen TA, Puska P, Gylling H, et al. Reduction of serum cholesterol with sitostanol-ester margarine in a mildly hypercholesterolemic population. *N Engl J Med*. 1995;333:1308–1312.

25. Blair SN, Capuzzi DM, Gottlieb SO, et al. Incremental reduction of serum total cholesterol and low-density lipoprotein cholesterol with the addition of plant stanol ester-containing spread to statin therapy. *Am J Cardiol*. 2000;86:46–52.

26. Moghadasian MH, Frohlich JJ. Effects of dietary phytosterols on cholesterol metabolism and atherosclerosis: clinical and experimental evidence. *Am J Med*. 1999;107: 588–594.

27. Williams CL, Bollella MC, Strobino BA, et al. Plant stanol ester and bran fiber in childhood: effects on lipids, stool weight and stool frequency in preschool children. *J Am Coll Nutr*. 1999;18:572–581.

28. Turnbull D, Whittaker MH, Frankos VH, et al. 13-week oral toxicity study with stanol esters in rats. *Regul Toxicol Pharmacol*. 1999;29(2 pt 1):216–226.

29. Nguyen TT, Dale LV, von Bergmann K, et al. Cholesterol-lowering effect of stanol ester in a US population of mildly hypercholesterolemic men and women: a randomized controlled trial. *Mayo Clin Proc*. 1999;74:1198–1206.

30. Gylling H, Miettinen TA. Cholesterol reduction by different plant stanol mixtures and with variable fat intake. *Metabolism*. 1999;48:575–580.

31. Tammi A, Ronnemaa T, Gylling H, et al. Plant stanol ester margarine lowers serum total and low-density lipoprotein cholesterol concentrations of healthy children: the STRIP project. Special Turku Coronary Risk Factors Intervention Project. *J Pediatr*. 2000;136:503–510.

32. Hallikainen MA, Sarkkinen ES, Uusitupa MI. Effects of low-fat stanol ester enriched margarines on concentrations of serum carotenoids in subjects with elevated serum cholesterol concentrations. *Eur J Clin Nutr*. 1999;53:966–969.

33. Miettinen TA, Puska P, Gylling H, et al. Reduction of serum cholesterol with sitostanol-ester margarine in a mildly hypercholesterolemic population. *N Engl J Med*. 1995;333:1308–1312.

34. Hallikainen MA, Sarkkinen ES, Uusitupa MI. Effects of low-fat stanol ester enriched margarines on concentrations of serum carotenoids in subjects with elevated serum cholesterol concentrations. *Eur J Clin Nutr*. 1999;53:966–969.

35. Anderson JW, Johnstone BM, Cook-Newell ME. Meta-analysis of the effects of soy protein intake on serum lipids. *N Engl J Med*. 1995;333:276–281.

36. Crouse JR III, Morgan T, Terry JG, et al. A randomized trial comparing the effect of casein with that of soy protein containing varying amounts of isoflavones on plasma concentrations of lipids and lipoproteins. *Arch Intern Med*. 1999;159:2070–2076.

37. Greaves KA, Parks JS, Williams JK, et al. Intact dietary soy protein, but not adding an isoflavone-rich soy extract to casein, improves plasma lipids in ovariectomized cynomolgus monkeys. *J Nutr*. 1999;129:1585–1592.

38. Simons LA, von Konigsmark M, Simons J, et al. Phyto-estrogens do not influence lipoprotein levels or endothelial function in healthy, postmenopausal women. *Am J Cardiol*. 2000;85:1297–1301.

39. Anderson JW, Johnstone BM, Cook-Newell ME. Meta-analysis of the effects of soy protein intake on serum lipids. *N Engl J Med*. 1995;333:276–281.

40. Divi RL, Chang HC, Doerge DR. Anti-thyroid isoflavones from soybean: isolation, characterization, and mechanisms of action. *Biochem Pharmacol*. 1997;54:1087–1096.

41. Chorazy PA, Himelhoch S, Hopwood NJ, et al. Persistent hypothyroidism in an infant receiving a soy formula: case report and review of the literature. *Pediatrics*. 1995;96(1 pt 1):148–150.

42. Jabbar MA, Larrea J, Shaw RA. Abnormal thyroid function tests in infants with congenital hypothyroidism: the influence of soy-based formula. *J Am Coll Nutr*. 1997;16:280–282.

43. Navert B, Sandstrom B, Cederblad A. Reduction of the phytate content of bran by leavening in bread and its effect on zinc absorption in man. *Br J Nutr*. 1985;53:47–53.

44. Hallberg L, Rossander L, Skanberg AB. Phytates and the inhibitory effects of bran on iron absorption in man. *Am J Clin Nutr*. 1987;45:988–996.

45. Heaney RP, Weaver CM, Fitzsimmons ML. Soybean phytate content: effect on calcium absorption. *Am J Clin Nutr*. 1991;53:745–747.

46. Vohra P, Gray GA, Kratzer FH. Phytic acid-metal complexes. *Proc Soc Exp Biol Med*. 1965;120:447–449.

47. Evans GW. Normal and abnormal zinc absorption in man and animals: the tryptophan connection. *Nutr Rev*. 1980; 38:137–141.

48. Crowell JA, Levine BS, Page JG, et al. Preclinical safety studies of isoflavones [abstract]. *J Nutr*. 2000;130(suppl): 677S.

49. [No authors listed]. Third International Symposium on the Role of Soy in Preventing and Treating Chronic Disease. October 31–November 3, 1999; Washington DC. Proceedings and abstracts. *J Nutr*. 2000;130(suppl):653S–711S.

50. Hilakivi-Clarke L, Cho E, Onojafe I, et al. Maternal exposure to genistein during pregnancy increases carcinogen-induced mammary tumorigenesis in female rat offspring. *Oncol Rep*. 1999;6:1089–1095.

51. Martini MC, Dancisak BB, Haggans CJ, et al. Effects of soy intake on sex hormone metabolism in premenopausal women. *Nutr Cancer*. 1999;34:133–139.

52. Scambia G, Mango D, Signorile PG, et al. Clinical effects of a standardized soy extract in postmenopausal women: a pilot study. *Menopause*. 2000;7:105–111.

53. Menendez R, Arruzazabala L, Mas R, et al. Cholesterol-lowering effect of policosanol on rabbits with hypercholesterolaemia induced by a wheat starch-casein diet. *Br J Nutr*. 1997;77:923–932.

54. Torres O, Agramonte AJ, Illnait J, et al. Treatment of hypercholesterolemia in NIDDM with policosanol. *Diabetes Care*. 1995;18:393–397.

55. Aneiros E, Mas R, Calderon B, et al. Effect of policosanol in lowering cholesterol levels in patients with type II hypercholesterolemia. *Curr Ther Res*. 1995;56:176–182.

56. Castano G, Canetti M, Moreira M, et al. Efficacy and tolerability of policosanol in elderly patients with type II hypercholesterolemia: a 12-month study. *Curr Ther Res*. 1995; 56:819–828.

57. Castano G, Tula L, Canetti M, et al. Effects of policosanol in hypertensive patients with type II hypercholesterolemia. *Curr Ther Res*. 1996;57:691–699.

58. Torres O, Agramonte AJ, Illnait J, et al. Treatment of hypercholesterolemia in NIDDM with policosanol. *Diabetes Care*. 1995;18:393–397.

59. Aneiros E, Calderon B, Mas R, et al. Effect of successive dose increases of policosanol on the lipid profile and tolerability of treatment. *Curr Ther Res*. 1993;54:304–312.

60. Castano G, Mas R, Nodarse M, et al. One-year study of the efficacy and safety of policosanol (5 mg twice daily) in the treatment of type II hypercholesterolemia. *Curr Ther Res*. 1995;56:296–304.

61. Batista J, Stusser R, Penichet M, et al. Doppler-ultrasound pilot study of the effects of long-term policosanol therapy on carotid-vertebral atherosclerosis. *Curr Ther Res*. 1995; 56:906–914.

62. Pons P, Rodriguez M, Mas R, et al. One-year efficacy and safety of policosanol in patients with type II hypercholesterolemia. *Curr Ther Res*. 1994;55:1084–1092.

63. Pons P, Rodriguez M, Robaina C, et al. Effects of successive dose increases of policosanol on the lipid profile of patients with type II hypercholesterolaemia and tolerability to treatment. *Int J Clin Pharm Res*. 1994;14:27–33.

64. Pons P, Mas R, Illnait J, et al. Efficacy and safety of policosanol in patients with primary hypercholesterolemia. *Curr Ther Res*. 1992;52:507–513.

65. Mas R, Castano G, Illnait J, et al. Effects of policosanol in patients with type II hypercholesterolemia and additional coronary risk factors. *Clin Pharmacol Ther*. 1999;65: 439–447.

66. Crespo N, Alvarez R, Mas R, et al. Effects of policosanol on patients with non-insulin-dependent diabetes mellitus and hypercholesterolemia: a pilot study. *Curr Ther Res*. 1997;58:44–51.

67. Castano G, Mas R, Fernandez L, et al. Effects of policosanol on postmenopausal women with type II hypercholesterolemia. *Gynecol Endocrinol*. 2000;14:187–195.

68. Benitez M, Romero C, Mas R, et al. A comparative study of policosanol versus pravastatin in patients with type II hypercholesterolemia. *Curr Ther Res*. 1997;58:859–867.

69. Ortensi G, Gladstein J, Valli H, et al. A comparative study of policosanol vs. simvastatin in elderly patients with hypercholesterolemia. *Curr Ther Res*. 1997;58:390–401.

70. Castano G, Mas R, Arruzazabala ML, et al. Effects of policosanol and pravastatin on lipid profile, platelet aggregation and endothelemia in older hypercholesterolemic patients. *Int J Clin Pharmacol Res*. 1999;19:105–116.

71. Crespo N, Illnait J, Mas R, et al. Comparative study of the efficacy and tolerability of policosanol and lovastatin in patients with hypercholesterolemia and noninsulin dependent diabetes mellitus. *Int J Clin Pharmacol Res*. 1999;19: 117–127.

72. Alcocer L, Fernandez L, Campos E, et al. A comparative study of policosanol versus acipimox in patients with type II hypercholesterolemia. *Int J Tissue React*. 1999;21:85–92.

73. Castano G, Mas R, Fernandez L, et al. Effects of policosanol on postmenopausal women with type II hypercholesterolemia. *Gynecol Endocrinol*. 2000;14:187–195.

74. Mas R, Castano G, Illnait J, et al. Effects of policosanol in patients with type II hypercholesterolemia and additional coronary risk factors. *Clin Pharmacol Ther*. 1999;65: 439–447.

75. Castano G, Mas R, Arruzazabala ML, et al. Effects of policosanol and pravastatin on lipid profile, platelet aggregation and endothelemia in older hypercholesterolemic patients. *Int J Clin Pharmacol Res*. 1999;19:105–116.

76. Crespo N, Illnait J, Mas R, et al. Comparative study of the efficacy and tolerability of policosanol and lovastatin in patients with hypercholesterolemia and noninsulin dependent diabetes mellitus. *Int J Clin Pharmacol Res*. 1999;19:117–127.

77. Alcocer L, Fernandez L, Campos E, et al. A comparative study of policosanol versus acipimox in patients with type II hypercholesterolemia. *Int J Tissue React*. 1999;21:85–92.

78. Benitez M, Romero C, Mas R, et al. A comparative study of policosanol versus pravastatin in patients with type II hypercholesterolemia. *Curr Ther Res*. 1997;58:859–867.

79. Ortensi G, Gladstein J, Valli H, et al. A comparative study of policosanol versus simvastatin in elderly patients with hypercholesterolemia. *Curr Ther Res*. 1997;58:390–401.

80. Torres O, Agramonte AJ, Illnait J, et al. Treatment of hypercholesterolemia in NIDDM with policosanol. *Diabetes Care*. 1995;18:393–397.

81. Crespo N, Alvarez R, Mas R, et al. Effects of policosanol on patients with non-insulin-dependent diabetes mellitus and hypercholesterolemia: a pilot study. *Curr Ther Res*. 1997;58:44–51.

82. Pons P, Rodriguez M, Mas R, et al. One-year efficacy and safety of policosanol in patients with type II hypercholesterolemia. *Curr Ther Res*. 1994;55:1084–1092.

83. Pons P, Mas R, Illnait J, et al. Efficacy and safety of policosanol in patients with primary hypercholesterolemia. *Curr Ther Res*. 1992;52:507–513.

84. Fernandez L, Mas R, Illnait J, et al. Policosanol: results of a postmarketing surveillance control on 27,879 patients. *Curr Ther Res*. 1998;59:717–722.

85. Rodriguez-Echenique C, Mesa R, Mas R, et al. Effects of policosanol chronically administered in male monkeys (*Macaca arctoides*). *Food Chem Toxicol*. 1994;32:565–575.

86. Mesa AR, Mas R, Noa M, et al. Toxicity of policosanol in beagle dogs: one-year study. *Toxicol Lett*. 1994;73:81–90.

87. Aleman CL, Mas R, Hernandez C, et al. A 12-month study of policosanol oral toxicity in Sprague Dawley rats. *Toxicol Lett*. 1994;70:77–87.

88. Rodriguez MD, Garcia H. Teratogenic and reproductive studies of policosanol in the rat and rabbit. *Teratog Carcinog Mutagen*. 1994;14:107–113.

89. Zardoya R, Tula L, Castano G, et al. Effects of policosanol on hypercholesterolemic abnormal serum biochemical indicators of hepatic function. *Curr Ther Res*. 1996;57:568–577.

90. Castano G, Tula L, Canetti M, et al. Effects of policosanol in hypertensive patients with type II hypercholesterolemia. *Curr Ther Res*. 1996;57:691–699.

91. Arruzazabala ML, Valdes S, Mas R, et al. Comparative study of policosanol, aspirin and the combination therapy policosanol-aspirin on platelet aggregation in healthy volunteers. *Pharmacol Res*. 1997;36:293–297.

92. Snider SR. Octacosanol in parkinsonism [letter]. *Ann Neurol.* 1984;16:723.

93. Heber D, Yip I, Ashley JM, et al. Cholesterol-lowering effects of a proprietary Chinese red-yeast-rice dietary supplement. *Am J Clin Nutr.* 1999;69:231–236.

94. Rippe J, Bonovich K, Colfer H, et al. A multi-center, self-controlled study of Cholestin™ in subjects with elevated cholesterol [abstract]. *Circulation.* 1999;99:1123.

95. Qin S, Zhang W, Qi P, et al. Elderly patients with primary hyperlipidemia benefited from treatment with a *Monascus purpureus* rice preparation: a placebo-controlled, double-blind clinical trial. Presented at: 39th Annual Conference on Cardiovascular Disease Epidemiology and Prevention; March 24–27, 1999; Orlando, Fla. Abstract P89.

96. Wang J, Lu Z, Chi J, et al. Multicenter clinical trial of the serum lipid-lowering effects of a *Monascus purpureus* (red yeast) rice preparation from traditional Chinese medicine. *Curr Ther Res.* 1997;58:964–978.

97. Chang M. *Cholestin™: Health-care Professional Product Guide.* Provo, Utah: Pharmanex; 1998: 1–6.

98. Ghirlanda G, Oradei A, Manto A, et al. Evidence of plasma CoQ10-lowering effect by HMG-CoA reductase inhibitors: a double-blind, placebo-controlled study. *J Clin Pharmacol.* 1993;33:226–229.

99. Mortensen SA, Leth A, Agner E, et al. Dose-related decrease of serum coenzyme Q10 during treatment with HMG-CoA reductase inhibitors. *Mol Aspects Med.* 1997; 18(suppl):S137–S144.

100. Folkers K, Langsjoen P, Willis R, et al. Lovastatin decreases coenzyme Q levels in humans. *Proc Natl Acad Sci U S A.* 1990;87:8931–8934.

101. Bargossi AM, Battino M, Gaddi A, et al. Exogenous CoQ10 preserves plasma ubiquinone levels in patients treated with 3-hydroxy-3-methylglutaryl coenzyme A reductase inhibitors. *Int J Clin Lab Res.* 1994;24:171–176.

102. Petrowicz O, Gebhardt R, Donner M, et al. Effects of artichoke leaf extract (ALE) on lipoprotein metabolism in vitro and in vivo [abstract]. *Atherosclerosis.* 1997;129:147.

103. Kraft K. Artichoke leaf extract—recent findings reflecting effects on lipid metabolism, liver and gastrointestinal tracts. *Phytomedicine*. 1997;4:369–378.

104. Englisch W, Beckers C, Unkauf M, et al. Efficacy of artichoke dry extract in patients with hyperlipoproteinemia. *Arzneimittelforschung*. 2000;50:260–265.

Chapter 5: Other Supplements for High Cholesterol

1. Singh V, Kaul S, Chander R, et al. Stimulation of low density lipoprotein receptor activity in liver membrane of guggulsterone treated rats. *Pharmacol Res*. 1990;22:37–44.

2. Singh RB, Niaz MA, Ghosh S. Hypolipidemic and antioxidant effects of *Commiphora mukul* as an adjunct to dietary therapy in patients with hypercholesterolemia. *Cardiovasc Drugs Ther*. 1994;8:659–664.

3. Verma SK, Bordia A. Effect of *Commiphora mukul* (gum guggulu) in patients of hyperlipidemia with special reference to HDL-cholesterol. *Indian J Med Res*. 1988;87: 356–360.

4. Nityanand S, Srivastava JS, Asthana OP. Clinical trials with gugulipid: A new hypolipidaemic agent. *J Assoc Physicians India*. 1989;37:323–328.

5. Gugulipid—six months toxicity data in rats and beagles. Central Drug Research Institute, Dossier, 8–58, 1982.

6. Gugulipid—Phase II clinical data. Central Drug Research Institute, Dossier, 5–8, 1981.

7. Gugulipid—six months toxicity data in rats and beagles. Central Drug Research Institute, Dossier, 8–58, 1982.

8. Nityanand S, Srivastava JS, Asthana OP. Clinical trials with gugulipid. A new hypolipidaemic agent. *J Assoc Physicians India*. 1989;37:323–328.

9. Singh RB, Niaz MA, Ghosh S. Hypolipidemic and antioxidant effects of *Commiphora mukul* as an adjunct to dietary therapy in patients with hypercholesterolemia. *Cardiovasc Drugs Ther*. 1994;8:659–664.

10. Agarwal RC, Singh SP, Saran RK, et al. Clinical trial of gugulipid—a new hyperlipidemic agent of plant origin in primary hyperlipidemia. *Indian J Med Res*. 1986;84:626–634.

11. Gaddi A, Descovich GC, Noseda G, et al. Controlled evaluation of pantethine, a natural hypolipidemic compound, in patients with different forms of hyperlipoproteinemia. *Atherosclerosis.* 1984;50:73–83.

12. Angelico M, Pinto G, Ciaccheri C, et al. Improvement in serum lipid profile in hyperlipoproteinaemic patients after treatment with pantethine: a crossover, double-blind trial versus placebo. *Curr Ther Res.* 1983;33:1091–1097.

13. Arsenio L, Caronna S, Lateana M, et al. Hyperlipidemia, diabetes and atherosclerosis: efficacy of treatment with pantethine [in Italian, English abstract]. *Acta Biomed Ateneo Parmense.* 1984;55:25–42.

14. Donati C, Barbi G, Cairo G, et al. Pantethine improves the lipid abnormalities of chronic hemodialysis patients: results of a multicenter clinical trial. *Clin Nephrol.* 1986;25:70–74.

15. Donati C, Bertieri RS, Barbi G. Pantethine, diabetes mellitus and atherosclerosis. Clinical study of 1045 patients [in Italian, English abstract]. *Clin Ter.* 1989;128:411–422.

16. Coronel F, Tornero F, Torrente J, et al. Treatment of hyperlipemia in diabetic patients on dialysis with a physiological substance. *Am J Nephrol.* 1991;11:32–36.

17. Carrara P, Matturri L, Galbussera M, et al. Pantethine reduces plasma cholesterol and the severity of arterial lesions in experimental hypercholesterolemic rabbits. *Atherosclerosis.* 1984;53:255–264.

18. Rubba R, Postiglione A, De Simone B, et al. Comparative evaluation of the lipid-lowering effects of fenofibrate and pantethine in type II hyperlipoproteinemia. *Curr Ther Res.* 1985;38:719–727.

19. Da Col PG, Cattin L, Fonda M, et al. Pantethine in the treatment of hypercholesterolemia: a randomized double-blind trial versus tiadenol. *Curr Ther Res.* 1984;36:314–322.

20. Arsenio L, Bodria P, Magnati G, et al. Effectiveness of long-term treatment with pantethine in patients with dyslipidemia. *Clin Ther.* 1986;8:537–545.

21. Qureshi AA, Bradlow BA, Salser WA, et al. Novel tocotrienols of rice bran modulate cardiovascular disease risk parameters of hypercholesterolemic humans. *J Nutr Biochem.* 1997;8:290–298.

22. Parker RA, Pearce BC, Clark RW, et al. Tocotrienols regulate cholesterol production in mammalian cells by post-transcriptional suppression of 3-hydroxy-3-methylglutaryl-coenzyme A reductase. *J Biol Chem.* 1993;268:11230–11238.

23. Tomeo AC, Geller M, Watkins TR, et al. Antioxidant effects of tocotrienols in patients with hyperlipidemia and carotid stenosis. *Lipids.* 1995;12:1179–1183.

24. Glore SR, Van Treeck D, Knehans AW, et al. Soluble fiber and serum lipids: a literature review. *J Am Diet Assoc.* 1994;94:425–436.

25. Maezaki Y, Tsuji K, Nakagawa Y, et al. Hypocholesterolemic effect of chitosan in adult males. *Biosci Biotechnol Biochem.* 1993;57:1439–1444.

26. Jing SB, Li L, Ji D, et al. Effect of chitosan on renal function in patients with chronic renal failure. *J Pharm Pharmacol.* 1997;49:721–723.

27. Ormrod D, Holmes CC, Miller TE. Dietary chitosan inhibits hypercholesterolaemia and atherogenesis in the apolipoprotein E-deficient mouse model of atherosclerosis. *Atherosclerosis.* 1998;138:329–334.

28. Deuchi K, Kanauchi O, Imasato Y, et al. Decreasing effect of chitosan on the apparent fat digestibility by rats fed on a high-fat diet. *Biosci Biotechnol Biochem.* 1994;58:1613–1616.

29. Deuchi K, Kanauchi O, Imasato Y, et al. Effect of the viscosity or deacetylation degree of chitosan on fecal fat excreted from rats fed on a high-fat diet. *Biosci Biotechnol Biochem.* 1995;59:781–785.

30. Deuchi K, Kanauchi O, Shizukuishi M, et al. Continuous and massive intake of chitosan affects mineral and fat-soluble vitamin status in rats fed on a high-fat diet. *Biosci Biotechnol Biochem.* 1995;59:1211–1216.

31. Kanauchi O, Deuchi K, Imasato Y, et al. Increasing effect of a chitosan and ascorbic acid mixture on fecal dietary fat excretion. *Biosci Biotechnol Biochem.* 1994;58:1617–1620.

32. Kobayashi T, Otsuka S, Yugari Y. Effect of chitosan on serum and liver cholesterol levels in cholesterol-fed rats. *Nutr Rep Int.* 1979;19:327–334.

33. Kanauchi O, Deuchi K, Imasato Y, et al. Increasing effect of a chitosan and ascorbic acid mixture on fecal dietary fat excretion. *Biosci Biotechnol Biochem*. 1994;58:1617–1620.

34. Koide SS. Chitin-chitosan: properties, benefits and risks. *Nutr Res*. 1998;18:1091–1101.

35. Deuchi K, Kanauchi O, Shizukuishi M, et al. Continuous and massive intake of chitosan affects mineral and fat-soluble vitamin status in rats fed on a high-fat diet. *Biosci Biotechnol Biochem*. 1995;59:1211–1216.

36. Koide SS. Chitin-chitosan: properties, benefits and risks. *Nutr Res*. 1998;18:1091–1101.

37. Harris WS. N-3 fatty acids and serum lipoproteins: human studies. *Am J Clin Nutr*. 1997;65(5 suppl):1645S–1654S.

38. Dyerberg J. N-3 fatty acids and coronary artery disease: potentials and problems. *Omega-3, Lipoproteins, and Atherosclerosis*. 1996;27:251–258. Cited by: Werbach MR. *Nutritional Influences on Illness* [book on CD-ROM]. Tarzana, Calif: Third Line Press; 1998.

39. Harris WS. N-3 fatty acids and serum lipoproteins: human studies. *Am J Clin Nutr*. 1997;65(5 suppl):1645S–1654S.

40. Harris WS. Dietary fish oil and blood lipids. *Curr Opin Lipidol*. 1996;7:3–7.

41. Cobiac L, Clifton PM, Abbey M, et al. Lipid, lipoprotein, and hemostatic effects of fish vs fish-oil n–3 fatty acids in mildly hyperlipidemic males. *Am J Clin Nutr*. 1991;53:1210–1216.

42. Montori VM, Farmer A, Wollan PC, et al. Fish oil supplementation in type 2 diabetes: a quantitative systematic review. *Diabetes Care*. 2000;23:1407–1415.

43. Laurora G, Cesarone MR, Belcaro G, et al. Control of the progress of arteriosclerosis in high risk subjects treated with mesoglycan. Measuring the intima media. *Minerva Cardioangiol*. 1998;46:41–47.

44. Tanganelli P, Bianciardi G, Carducci A, et al. Updating on in-vivo and in-vitro effects of heparin and other glycosaminoglycans (mesoglycan) on arterial endothelium: a morphometrical study. *Int J Tissue React*. 1992;14:149–153.

45. Morrison LM, Enrick N. Coronary heart disease: reduction of death rate by chondroitin sulfate A. *Angiology.* 1973; 24:269–287.

46. Nakazawa K, Murata K. The therapeutic effect of chondroitin polysulphate in elderly atherosclerotic patients. *J Int Med Res.* 1978;6:217–225.

47. Saba P, Galeone F, Giuntoli F, et al. Hypolipidemic effect of mesoglycan in hyperlipidemic patients. *Curr Ther Res.* 1986;40:761–768.

48. Davini P, Bigalli A, Lamanna F, et al. Controlled study on L-carnitine therapeutic efficacy in post-infarction. *Drugs Exp Clin Res.* 1992;18:355–365.

49. Oosthuizen W, Vorster HH, Vermaak WJ, et al. Lecithin has no effect on serum lipoprotein, plasma fibrinogen and macro molecular protein complex levels in hyperlipidaemic men in a double-blind controlled study. *Eur J Clin Nutr.* 1998;52:419–424.

50. Roeback JR Jr, Hla KM, Chambless LE, et al. Effects of chromium supplementation on serum high-density lipoprotein cholesterol levels in men taking beta-blockers. A randomized, controlled trial. *Ann Intern Med*. 1991;115: 917–924.

51. Babu JR, Sundravel S, Arumugam G, et al. Salubrious effect of vitamin C and vitamin E on tamoxifen-treated women in breast cancer with reference to plasma lipid and lipoprotein levels. *Cancer Lett*. 2000;151:1–5.

52. Earnest CP, Almada AL, and Mitchell TL. High-performance capillary electrophoresis-pure creatine monohydrate reduces blood lipids in men and women. *Clin Sci (Colch)*. 1996;91:113–118.

53. Bell L, Halstenson CE, Halstenson CJ, et al. Cholesterol-lowering effects of calcium carbonate in patients with mild to moderate hypercholesterolemia. *Arch Intern Med*. 1992;152:2441–2444.

54. Bostick RM, Fosdick L, Grandits GA, et al. Effect of calcium supplementation on serum cholesterol and blood pressure: a randomized, double-blind, placebo-controlled, clinical trial. *Arch Fam Med*. 2000;9:31–39.

55. Agerholm-Larsen L, Raben A, Haulrik N, et al. Effect of 8 week intake of probiotic milk products on risk factors for cardiovascular diseases. *Eur J Clin Nutr*. 2000;54:288–297.

56. Agerbaek M, Gerdes LU, Richelsen B. Hypocholesterol-aemic effect of a new fermented milk product in healthy middle-aged men. *Eur J Clin Nutr*. 1995;49:346–352.

57. Bertolami MC, Faludi AA, Batlouni M. Evaluation of the effects of a new fermented milk product (Gaio) on primary hypercholesterolemia. *Eur J Clin Nutr*. 1999;53:97–101.

58. Richelsen B, Kristensen K, Pedersen SB. Long-term (6 months) effect of a new fermented milk product on the level of plasma lipoproteins—a placebo-controlled and double blind study. *Eur J Clin Nutr*. 1996;50:811–815.

59. Anderson JW, Gilliland SE. Effect of fermented milk (yo-gurt) containing *Lactobacillus acidophilus* L1 on serum cholesterol in hypercholesterolemic humans. *J Am Coll Nutr*. 1999;18:43–50.

60. Iwata K, Inayama T, Kato T. Effects of *Spirulina platensis* on plasma lipoprotein lipase activity in fructose-induced hyperlipidemic rats. *J Nutr Sci Vitaminol (Tokyo)*. 1990; 36:165–171.

61. Gonzalez de Rivera C, Miranda-Zamora R, Diaz-Zagoya JC, et al. Preventive effect of *Spirulina maxima* on the fatty liver induced by a fructose-rich diet in the rat, a prelimi-nary report. *Life Sci*. 1993;53:57–61.

62. Nakaya N, Homma Y, Goto Y. Cholesterol lowering effect of *Spirulina*. *Nutr Rep Int*. 1988;37:1329–1337.

63. Story JA, LePage SL, Petro MS, et al. Interactions of alfalfa plant and sprout saponins with cholesterol in vitro and in cholesterol-fed rats. *Am J Clin Nutr*. 1984;39:917–929.

64. Malinow MR, McLaughlin P, Naito HK, et al. Effect of al-falfa meal on shrinkage (regression) of atherosclerotic plaques during cholesterol feeding in monkeys. *Atheroscle-rosis*. 1978;30:27–43.

65. Malinow MR, Connor WE, McLaughlin P, et al. Choles-terol and bile acid balance in *Macaca fascicularis*. Effects of alfalfa saponins. *J Clin Invest*. 1981;67:156–162.

66. Esper E, Barichello AW, Chan EK, et al. Synergistic lipid-lowering effects of alfalfa meal as an adjuvant to the partial ileal bypass operation. *Surgery*. 1987;102:39–51.

67. Dixit VP, Joshi SC. Antiatherosclerotic effects of alfalfa meal ingestion in chicks: a biochemical evaluation. *Indian J Physiol Pharmacol*. 1985;29:47–50.

68. Malinow MR, McLaughlin P, Papworth L, et al. Effect of alfalfa saponins on intestinal cholesterol absorption in rats. *Am J Clin Nutr*. 1977;30:2061–2067.

69. Malinow MR, McLaughlin P, Stafford C, et al. Comparative effects of alfalfa saponins and alfalfa fiber on cholesterol absorption in rats. *Am J Clin Nutr*. 1979;32:1810–1812.

70. Malinow MR, McLaughlin P, Stafford C, et al. Alfalfa saponins and alfalfa seeds. Dietary effects in cholesterol-fed rabbits. *Atherosclerosis*. 1980;37:433–438.

71. Yanaura S, Sakamoto M. Effect of alfalfa meal on experimental hyperlipidemia [in Japanese; English abstract]. *Nippon Yakurigaku Zasshi*. 1975;71:387–393.

72. Srinivasan SR, Patton D, Radhakrishnamurthy B, et al. Lipid changes in atherosclerotic aortas of *Macaca fascicularis* after various regression regimens. *Atherosclerosis*. 1980;37:591–601.

73. Malinow MR. Experimental models of atherosclerosis regression. *Atherosclerosis*. 1983;48:105–118.

74. Malinow MR, Connor WE, McLaughlin P, et al. Cholesterol and bile acid balance in *Macaca fascicularis*. Effects of alfalfa saponins. *J Clin Invest*. 1981;67:156–162.

75. Molgaard J, von Schenck H, Olsson AG. Alfalfa seeds lower low density lipoprotein cholesterol and apolipoprotein B concentrations in patients with type II hyperlipoproteinemia. *Atherosclerosis*.1987;65:173–179.

76. Malinow MR, McLaughlin P, Stafford C. Alfalfa seeds: effects on cholesterol metabolism. *Experientia*. 1980;36:562–564.

Chapter 6: Lifestyle Changes

1. Truswell AS, Choudhury N. Monounsaturated oils do not all have the same effect on plasma cholesterol. *Eur J Clin Nutr*. 1998;52:312–315.

2. Kris-Etherton PM, Yu S. Individual fatty acid effects on plasma lipids and lipoproteins: human studies. *Am J Clin Nutr.* 1997;65(5 suppl):1628S–1644S.

3. Clarke R, Frost C, Collins R, et al. Dietary lipids and blood cholesterol: quantitative meta-analysis of metabolic ward studies. *BMJ.* 1997;314:112–117.

4. Tang JL, Armitage JM, Lancaster T, et al. Systematic review of dietary intervention trials to lower total blood cholesterol in free-living subjects. *BMJ.* 1998;316:1213–1220.

5. Hu FB, Stampfer MJ, Manson JE, et al. Frequent nut consumption and risk of coronary heart disease in women: prospective cohort study. *BMJ.* 1998;317:1341–1345.

6. Fraser GE, Sabate J, Beeson WL, et al. A possible protective effect of nut consumption on risk of coronary heart disease. The Adventist Health Study. *Arch Intern Med.* 1992;152:1416–1424.

7. Abbey M, Noakes M, Belling GB, et al. Partial replacement of saturated fatty acids with almonds or walnuts lowers total plasma cholesterol and low-density-lipoprotein cholesterol. *Am J Clin Nutr.* 1994;59:995–999.

8. Spiller GA, Jenkins DA, Bosello O, et al. Nuts and plasma lipids: an almond-based diet lowers LDL-C while preserving HDL-C. *J Am Coll Nutr.* 1998;17:285–290.

9. Spiller GA, Jenkins DJ, Cragen LN, et al. Effect of a diet high in monounsaturated fat from almonds on plasma cholesterol and lipoproteins. *J Am Coll Nutr.* 1992;11:126–130.

10. Curb JD, Wergowske G, Dobbs JC, et al. Serum lipid effects of a high-monounsaturated fat diet based on macadamia nuts. *Arch Intern Med.* 2000;160:1154–1158.

11. Zambon D, Sabate J, Munoz S, et al. Substituting walnuts for monounsaturated fat improves the serum lipid profile of hypercholesterolemic men and women. A randomized crossover trial. *Ann Intern Med.* 2000;132:538–546.

12. Morgan WA, Clayshulte BJ. Pecans lower low-density lipoprotein cholesterol in people with normal lipid levels. *J Am Diet Assoc.* 2000;100:312–318.

13. Mensink RP, Katan MB. Effect of dietary trans fatty acids on high-density and low-density lipoprotein cholesterol levels in healthy subjects. *N Engl J Med.* 1990;323:439–445.

14. Sundram K, Ismail A, Hayes KC, et al. Trans (elaidic) fatty acids adversely affect the lipoprotein profile relative to specific saturated fatty acids in humans. *J Nutr.* 1997;127: 514S–520S.

15. Kummerow FA, Zhou Q, Mahfouz MM. Effects of trans fatty acids on calcium influx into human arterial endothelial cells. *Am J Clin Nutr.* 1999;70:832–838.

16. Davidson MH, Maki KC, Kong JC, et al. Long-term effects of consuming foods containing psyllium seed husk on serum lipids in subjects with hypercholesterolemia. *Am J Clin Nutr.* 1998;67:367–376.

17. Gerhardt AL, Gallo NB. Full-fat rice bran and oat bran similarly reduce hypercholesterolemia in humans. *J Nutr.* 1998;128:865–869.

18. Goel V, Ooraikul B, Basu TK. Cholesterol lowering effects of rhubarb stalk fiber in hypercholesterolemic men. *J Am Coll Nutr.* 1997;16:600–604.

19. Sprecher DL, Harris BV, Goldberg AC, et al. Efficacy of psyllium in reducing serum cholesterol levels in hypercholesterolemic patients on high or low-fat diets. *Ann Intern Med.* 1993;119(7 pt 1):545–554.

20. Schuit AJ, Schouten EG, Miles TP, et al. The effect of six months training on weight, body fatness and serum lipids in apparently healthy elderly Dutch men and women. *Int J Obes Relat Metab Disord.* 1998;22:847–853.

21. Dengel DR, Hagberg JM, Pratley RE, et al. Improvements in blood pressure, glucose metabolism and lipoprotein lipids after aerobic exercise plus weight loss in obese, hypertensive middle-aged men. *Metabolism.* 1998;47: 1075–1082.

22. Erikssen G, Liestol K, Bjornholt J, et al. Changes in physical fitness and changes in mortality. *Lancet.* 1998;352:759–762.

23. Leon AS, Myers MJ, Connett J. Leisure time physical activity and the 16-year risks of mortality from coronary heart disease and all-causes in the Multiple Risk Factor Intervention Trial (MRFIT). *Int J Sports Med.* 1997;18(suppl 3):S208–S215.

24. Klatsky AL, Armstrong MA, Friedman GD. Alcohol and mortality. *Ann Intern Med.* 1992;117:646–654.

25. Steinberg D, Pearson TA, Kuller LH. Alcohol and atherosclerosis. *Ann Intern Med*. 1991;114:967–976.

26. Constant J. Alcohol, ischemic heart disease, and the French paradox. *Coron Artery Dis*. 1997;8:645–649.

27. Schwarz B, Bischof HP, Kunze M. Coffee, tea, and lifestyle. *Prev Med*. 1994;23:377–384.

28. Ornish D, Brown SE, Scherwitz LW, et al. Can lifestyle changes reverse coronary heart disease? The Lifestyle Heart Trial. *Lancet*. 1990;336:129–133.

Chapter 7:
Conventional Treatment for High Cholesterol

1. Kjekshus J, Pedersen TR. Reducing the risk of coronary events: evidence from the Scandinavian Simvastatin Survival Study. *Am J Cardiol*. 1995;76:64C–68C.

2. Sacks FM, Pfeffer MA, Moye LA, et al. The effect of pravastatin on coronary events after myocardial infarction in patients with average cholesterol levels. Cholesterol and Recurrent Events Trial Investigators. *N Engl J Med*. 1996; 335:1001–1009.

3. Downs JR, Clearfield M, Weis S, et al. Primary prevention of acute coronary events with lovastatin in men and women with average cholesterol levels. *JAMA*. 1998;279: 1615–1622.

4. *Physicians' Desk Reference*. Montvale, NJ: Medical Economics Co; 1998:938.

5. Ghirlanda G, Oradei A, Manto A, et al. Evidence of plasma CoQ10-lowering effect by HMG-CoA reductase inhibitors: a double-blind, placebo-controlled study. *J Clin Pharmacol*. 1993;33:226–229.

6. Bargossi AM, Grossi G, Fiorella PL, et al. Exogenous CoQ10 supplementation prevents plasma ubiquinone reduction induced by HMG-CoA reductase inhibitors. *Mol Aspects Med*. 1994;15(suppl):S187–S193.

7. Frick MH, Elo O, Haapa K, et al. Helsinki Heart Study: primary-prevention trial with gemfibrozil in middle-aged men with dyslipidemia. Safety of treatment, changes in risk factors, and incidence of coronary heart disease. *N Engl J Med*. 1987;317:1237–1245.

8. *Physicians' Desk Reference*. Montvale, NJ: Medical Economics Co; 1998:2107.

9. *Physicians' Desk Reference*. Montvale, NJ: Medical Economics Co; 1998:2108.

Index

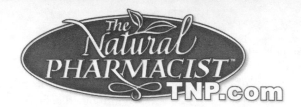

About the Author

Darin Ingels, N.D., is a graduate of Bastyr University and a licensed naturopathic physician. He is also a certified medical technologist and has been involved in medical education for more than eight years. Dr. Ingels currently practices in Seattle and continues to lecture extensively to health care professionals and the public. He lives in Kirkland, Washington, with his wife, Michelle.

About the Series Editors

Steven Bratman, M.D., is Medical Director of TNP.com and Senior Editor for all online content. Dr. Bratman is both a strong proponent and vocal critic of alternative treatment, and he believes that alternative medicine has both strengths and weaknesses, just like conventional medicine. His books include *The Alternative Medicine Sourcebook: A Realistic Evaluation of Alternative Healing Methods* (1997), *The Alternative Medicine Ratings Guide: An Expert Panel Ranks the Best Alternative Treatments for Over 80 Conditions* (Prima Health, 1998), the professional text *Clinical Evaluation of Medicinal Herbs and Other Therapeutic Natural Products* (Prima Health, 1999), and the following titles in THE NATURAL PHARMACIST™ series: *Your Complete Guide to Herbs* (Prima Health, 1999), *Your Complete Guide to Illnesses and Their Natural Remedies* (Prima Health, 1999), *The Natural Health Bible, Revised and Expanded 2nd Edition* (Prima Health, 2000), and *Treating Depression* (Prima Health, 1999).

David J. Kroll, Ph.D., is a professor of pharmacology and toxicology at the University of Colorado School of Pharmacy and a consultant for pharmacists, physicians, and alternative practitioners on the indications and cautions for herbal medicine use. He received a degree in toxicology from the Philadelphia College of Pharmacy and Science and obtained his Ph.D. from the University of Florida College of Medicine. Dr. Kroll has lectured widely and has published articles in a number of medical journals, abstracts, and newsletters.